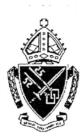

# KING ALFRED'S COLLEGE
# WINCHESTER
Library: 01962 827306

**To be returned on or before the day
marked below, subject to recall**

# Opening Up Care

# Opening Up Care

## ACHIEVING PRINCIPLED PRACTICE IN HEALTH AND SOCIAL CARE INSTITUTIONS

David Stanley BPhil, PhD, CRCCYP, SCRCCYP

*Head, Division of Primary Health and Adult & Community Studies/Co-director, Centre for the Care of Older People,*
*University of Northumbria at Newcastle, UK*

and

Jan Reed BA, RN, PhD

*Professor of Health Care for Older People/Co-director, Centre for the Care of Older People,*
*University of Northumbria at Newcastle, UK*

A member of the Hodder Headline Group
LONDON • SYDNEY • AUCKLAND

First published in Great Britain in 1999 by
Arnold, a member of the Hodder Headline Group,
338 Euston Road, London NW1 3BH

**http://www.arnoldpublishers.com**

© 1999 David Stanley and Jan Reed

*British Library Cataloguing in Publication Data*
A catalogue record for this book is available from the British Library

ISBN 0 340 70591 4 (pb)

1 2 3 4 5 6 7 8 9 10

Commissioning Editor: Cathy Peck
Production Editor: Liz Gooster
Production Controller: Iain McWilliams
Project Manager: Paula O'Connell
Cover Design: Mouse Mat

Typeset in 10 on 12 Palatino by Phoenix Photosetting, Chatham, Kent
Printed and bound in Great Britain by JW Arrowsmith Ltd, Bristol

What do you think about this book? Or any other Arnold title?
Please send your comments to feedback.arnold@hodder.co.uk

# Contents

# Preface

The subtitle of this book calls for some degree of explanation. We feel strongly that much of the interest in institutional care, especially in the literature, is directed at the institution as a private, if not secretive, world. However, our own experiences of working in and around those very same institutions made us conscious of a need to demonstrate that those characteristics of 'institutionalisation' which are so often identified as the responsibility of others are, on the contrary, the responsibilities of us all. We wanted to 'open up' those experiences to scrutiny, partly because private problems only ever lead to private solutions, and there is too much evidence to indicate anything other than the inadequacy of such a reliance. Mostly, however, we wanted to 'open up' care in institutions because we believe that it can help us to improve the quality of its delivery by underpinning practice with clearly articulated principles. We wanted to write a text aimed with a primary focus at social and health care students at professional and post-qualification training levels. We hope, therefore, that it will be read by students, practitioners and researchers who operate in these sectors. We would also like to think that the book will be of value to other stakeholders and users of the residential health and social care services.

The book itself reflects our own personal–professional journeys: journeys which we felt were worth exploring and sharing. In both thinking about and illustrating our points, we have reflected upon our own experiences of practice, research and teaching. We acknowledge that there might exist a tension in moving between research on practice and inventories on good practice requirements. Much of the former is depressing and without positive contribution to practice, and, whilst we feel that there may be no shortage of the latter, they do not necessarily offer systems, processes or positive models of implementation. We also acknowledge both the paradox and the danger of setting out to present the very same material and believing that we can do it in a different and, by our own definition, more effective way. The paradox is that we use the same framework, though to different ends; and the danger lies in the possibility that we fail to achieve our goals. We are content to leave it to the readers to judge the result for themselves.

We shall be introducing a broad range of theoretical perspectives across an equally broad range of disciplines. There is a necessary expectation that the reader will approach this book with some degree of existing awareness of the perspectives which it addresses, whether such awareness be historical, experiential or theoretical. Whilst some of the material will, therefore, be familiar to the reader, we revisit it for particular purposes. We are constantly reminded that it is unsafe to assume, for example, a universal familiarity with Goffman's (1961) *Asylums*, for there are new generations of practitioners and students who, whilst they might have heard of that well-known name, will not necessarily have studied the text in detail. Similarly, where we have given a synoptic introduction to broad approaches, for example management theory or values and ethics, we have done so on the basis that it makes more sense within our structure to present a coherent package of material, in relation to our developing discussions, than to assume that the reader is either familiar with it or is able easily to locate alternative sources. Few will disagree with the notion of grounding practice in theory and, of course, vice versa, but all too often we may wrongly assume an adequate theory base.

As we weave our way amongst the pragmatic, the professional and the ideological, and between thinking about situations and offering solutions, we hope that our own perspectives will offer a contribution to the development of effective, positive practice. In Chapter 4, when writing about translating our values into practice, we comment that 'it is part of our aspiration to encourage the reader positively to apply these values, rather than simply to know them' (p. 54). In similar vein, we present this book as a vehicle for encouraging both the thinking about *and* development of individuals' own particular contributions to, and experiences of, the institutional setting, whether this be as a service-user, practitioner, student, or researcher. Our subject is a difficult one and its practice is as demanding a job as we can imagine, but it also has the capacity to be immensely rewarding.

Chapters 1 and 2 introduce the contexts of institutional care, explaining why we have chosen to use the much discredited 'I' word, and go on to explore current debates, all with a focus on implications for practice. Chapters 3, 4, 5 and 6 identify a range of fundamental issues and examine a number of quite discrete models in order to develop key perspectives. Some of the book, for example Chapter 4, leans heavily on theories of management and quality, whilst other parts, for example Chapter 5, are more concerned with developing an open discussion. Chapters 7 and 8 are designed to move our thinking forward into producing an active response to all of this material. We develop the notion of an ethical audit, by which we mean a model of transforming thinking into action, thereby making a positive contribution to the structures – physical, emotional and environmental – which serve to shape the lived experiences of institutional care.

# Context setting

Introduction

The 'I' word and the power of language

Historical antecedents – an overview

## Introduction

There will not be a reader of this book whose life has not, in a multitude of ways, been profoundly touched by his or her personal experiences of institutions. Many of us began life in one by virtue of a hospital delivery; we were, by and large, nurtured in the institution that is the family; we all spent formative years – and some of us continue to spend adult years – in the various forms of educational institutions; and many of us then go on to work in other, equally varied forms, of institutions. There are conceptual, abstract institutions, such as the family, which do not have walls but can, on the one hand, exert incredible control over lives and, at the other extreme, can fail to fulfil its function by not imposing boundaries on its members. Then there are institutions which are instantly recognisable by their grim walls as state organs of control: old style psychiatric hospitals, prisons, and new but equally forbidding secure units. Geographical location alone is not a key indicator to the status of an institution, but location and physical appearance alone can often yield external clues to the internal environment. In yet another sense we talk of financial institutions – banks, building societies – or the institutions of government such as the Houses of Parliament and the Civil Service. However, what we are specifically concerned with here is to explore ideas and examples of those institutions which, loosely speaking, comprise the care-oriented health and welfare services which exist within our society.

These services defy easy definition or neat categorisation. Our particular focus is on the residential and nursing institutions of social and health care, and it is in this sense that we have an interest in the word 'institution'. However, this book is ultimately concerned with what goes on inside institutions, and that activity is known by a wide range of generic descriptors. Residential care, nursing care, health care, social care, group care and group living are all terms which occur, each of them representing a particular construction of meaning as understood by their users, partly as a consequence of their experiential backgrounds or professional origins. It is through the exemplars to which we shall refer that we hope to develop a taxonomy of institutions and their associated language, which will illustrate our fundamental belief that it is as important to examine the broader nature of institutions as it is to focus on the specific activities that go on within them. Moreover, at a time when the imperatives of interdisciplinary, multi-professional working are increasingly valued, it is essential to build bridges which will help us to make the links between what have, until relatively recently, been seen substantively as discrete working environments. We have been motivated to write this book as a result of our own discovery of the connections between our very different practice backgrounds – social work and nursing. In acknowledging the fact that joint working, and the developing initiatives for joint training, are at the forefront of much practice development, we also recognise the need for material which brings together these various dimensions.

## The 'I' word and the power of language

Those who have got as far as opening the first pages of this book will have done so for a variety of reasons, and with a range of expectations. The common experience, however, will have been reading the title on the cover, which contains words which have evoked certain images and ideas. When trying to think of a title for this book we were aware of the power of words and, obviously because we wanted a lot of people to read it, we were concerned about evoking images and ideas which were exciting and appealing, rather than gloomy and depressing. This, however, was very difficult to do – one commentator suggested that we should not use the word 'institution' even though that was, essentially, what the book was about, because it would 'put people off'. This put us in something of a dilemma – should we try to think of a more acceptable euphemism for institutional care, and then spring the idea on the readers once they had got well into the book? Or should we be fairly upfront and have the 'I' word on the cover, and risk not attracting readers who found it too depressing?

We decided to be upfront and use the 'I' word in the subtitle, against such marketing advice, partly because we felt that readers should know what they were buying, but also because the debate itself felt like an example of some of the problems that we wanted to explore, and which we feel contribute to the problems of delivering care and services in places known as institutions. If the word on the cover of a book can stop people wanting to read it or buy it, what does that word say to people who live or work in institutions? If the place that you go to for help and support is described as 'an institution', how do you feel about the care you receive? If the place where you work is called 'an institution', how do you feel about the work that you do?

In a world in which words simply serve as ways of precisely labelling things, we could argue that the term institution is simply a technical term, and does not carry any negative or positive connotations – it is a descriptive word in much the same way as 'cat', 'dog', or 'plant pot' are. We do not live in this world, however, and words do much more than simply label things – the labels evoke feelings and ideas, and refer to sets of values (Reed and Ground,

1997). The word 'institution' then, in modern day language, is often a derogatory term and refers not just to a type of care setting, but also to the discredited activities that are *thought to* go on in it – it has an evaluative role.

It is important, however, to emphasise the phrase 'thought to' in this last sentence, because it points to another way in which words work – they do not simply reflect ideas and values, but they can shape and reinforce them. If the word 'institution' is used as a shorthand term for a range of activities (incarceration, routinisation, dehumanisation) of which we disapprove, and if it is applied in a cavalier fashion to a range of care settings, then it becomes easy to assume that everything that we call an institution will exhibit these characteristics, even if a more careful examination might reveal that they do not. Such shorthand use, then, because people assume its accuracy, does not prompt critical evaluation of the things it describes – we can all carry on comfortable in the confidence that we can all spot an institution when we see one, and that we all know what goes on in them.

The power of words to perpetuate and reinforce stereotypes and assumptions is perhaps the best place to start in a discussion of institutional care, because most people will come to this discussion with some images and ideas firmly established, and these will colour and shape their thinking in many subtle and not so subtle ways. If we are to get anywhere at all in developing and re-thinking institutional care, then we need to begin by re-thinking the way in which we respond to and communicate ideas about institutions. Examining our language and the words that we use is one way of exploring our position on things, working out how we arrive there and deciding where we want to go next.

## LAY TALK AND EVERYDAY LANGUAGE

Perhaps the best type of language to start with is 'lay talk', i.e. the everyday language that people with no pretensions to expert knowledge use in conversation. Such talk is, however, difficult to capture in any systematic way, partly because its ordinariness makes it difficult to notice, and also because it is often so fluid and complex – changing rapidly over time and across groups. What we can do here, however, is to think through some examples of lay talk about institutions and map out how they may impinge upon our thinking.

Possibly the best place to start this is with a joke, humour being one way in which ideas are communicated and shaped. Perhaps one of the best known, or most familiar, jokes about institutions goes like this:

Marriage is a great institution – for those who like institutions!

This joke appeals to and plays on conflicts between the meanings of the word institution, first the approving use to describe things that are valued highly, a sort of 'official', slightly pompous use of the term, and second the other meaning, shared by the audience, which is the critical use of the term to delineate things that are restrictive, repressive and unpleasant, and which only very strange people would like. In this way the joke manages to do several things. It mocks the orthodox or official view of society about institutions as 'good things', it points out the alternative view of institutions as 'bad things', and it encourages us to draw conclusions about those people who adopt the first view – that they are odd, and not like us, the audience.

One joke, of course, cannot sum up an entire culture, but the success of this one (it seems to have been around a long time, although its origins are impossible to pinpoint exactly) suggests that it has some resonance with those who hear it. What it alerts us to is the approval with which anti-institutionalism is met, but perhaps we should also think about the position that the joke attacks – the view that institutions are 'good things'.

The use of the word 'institution' in an approving sense is also found in lay talk, though perhaps mainly in periods earlier than our own. In the North East, for example, it is common to see the words 'Miners' Institute', one form of the root word, engraved over the doorways of libraries and recreational centres built for miners around the turn of the nineteenth century. Given that the policy was, presumably, to encourage people to use these facilities rather than to put them off, we can infer that the term did not have the negative associations that it always seems to have now. What it does seem to confer is a recognition or formalisation of things that otherwise could be thought of as casual or *ad hoc*. The Miners' Institute is not just a collection of miners playing football on waste ground or lending each other books, but it is something that is organised and regularised and acknowledged to be important. Interestingly, a similar process seems to go on in academic circles, where disparate groups of researchers doing idiosyncratic research decide to come together and call themselves an institute, immediately implying a degree of cohesion and gravitas which may not have been apparent before.

Formalising things is, however, a double-edged sword. It may well have the effect of recognising activities, affording them more respect and perhaps organising them more efficiently, but other aspects to becoming an institution can be seen in a less favourable light. Spontaneity may be lost, regulation may stifle innovation, and the individual is subsumed to the collective will. The people whose recreation is organised by an institute may long for the days of playing football on waste land.

Similar ambiguities of feeling are reflected in other ways in which the term 'institution' is used in a complimentary way. Financial institutions, for example, employ the language of economic and political power, with its associated high status. In the main, financial institutions are highly regarded, but there are also those of quite dubious reputation, either because of their shady dealings or the unmitigated greed they display. When we talk about financial institutions, then, we can be simultaneously acknowledging the power and respectability that they have and the disdain with which they are sometimes viewed. Sometimes this ambiguity is reflected in the differences we identify within a type of institution. For example, the institutions which we use in a normative way – mainstream schools and universities, acute hospital services – are on the whole associated with normative language. We talk of these institutions in ways that suggest that they are to be admired, or at the very least accepted as a sensible way of dealing with various societal activities. Where institutions deal with problems or people who are not 'normal', however (for example those institutions which deal in 'social problems' rather than purely general health, or educational difficulties rather than educational progression), problems are quite often presented through language which emphasises marginalisation and negativity. The term institution here carries a derogatory sense.

It is not sufficient, therefore, to talk generically about language as if it were stratified only in one way – things are much more complex than this. The above examples have a range of lexicons associated with them. In the main, financial institutions have high status, although they can also be reviled. In the main, schools are seen as desirable, progressive institutions of society, political expediency and dogma notwithstanding (and the notion of residential schooling, in its boarding sense, has a special social standing), although our personal experience of them may be negative. Both of these instances are heavily represented by examples to which many people would aspire: the public school and the centre of commerce. Conversely, the residential institutions of social welfare which address social problems not considered normative or mainstream have an associated vocabulary and meaning which serves to pathologise as much as it serves to explain. The term 'special', when applied to some things, can convey approval or desirability, but when applied to a school can be taken as a euphemism for a place which deals with those who are not valued by society.

It is also interesting to note that the mechanisms and processes which can be found within institutions are often quite different in value terms from the sums of their parts. The brutalising behaviour which is associated with prison life can often be found, perhaps at different levels and manifested through different dynamics, in elite boarding schools. Similarly the depersonalisation, objectification and batch treatment characteristics which have been identified as fundamentals of the 'total' institution can be found in settings which are valued by, rather than marginalised in, our society, such as the religious institution, the military academy and the football club.

What all of this means for us within the context of this book is that the arena into which we are looking is subtle and sophisticated, blunt and crude, generalised and specific in equal turns. It is precisely because of this complexity that different languages and different interpretations of these languages have developed to enable participants in the situation to address the wide range of perceptions and functions. Too often we see the world of the institution solely from our own experiences within it. If we are to be effective professional workers – or even if we wish merely to be informed – then we also have a duty to understand how others, particularly those who are served by institutions, see their experience of that world. Understanding the different ways of talking about institutions helps us to see how our practice is shaped by this talk.

## DICTIONARY DEFINITIONS

Lay talk is, as we have said, difficult to capture, but one device for doing so is the dictionary, which records the use of words and the meanings attributed to them. The record is not merely the most common or prominent uses of words, but aims to cover the whole range of usage, and it therefore provides a broader view of language and ideas. Moreover, looking at the dictionary record of a word's use or meaning can also give some sense of the change of usage over time, in the description of archaic forms, or of the Latin or Greek roots of the word. When we look at a dictionary entry on the word 'institution' therefore, we can expand upon an informal exploration of lay talk by looking at uses which are not common, or which have fallen out of use, and in doing so widen our ideas about what the word can mean.

The *Collins English Dictionary* (1991) gives eight definitions of institution, some of which are quite specialised (such as ecclesiastical terminology). Interestingly the first definition given is 'the act of instituting', in other words the use of the word as a verb. This explicit reference to action comes as quite a surprise if one's ideas about institutions do not extend to thinking about processes or the activity involved in setting them up – if the institution is only thought of as something that already exists. Yet the use of institution as a verb should point us to considering institutions as things that were created by social activity, rather than as almost permanent features of the landscape.

The second definition, 'an organisation or establishment founded for a specific purpose, such as a hospital, church or college', perhaps matches more closely the usual use of the word to describe a setting for care. What it does not do, however, is perform any evaluative function – it is a neutral definition which does not make any suggestion about whether such things are regarded positively or negatively. If we expect the term to be accompanied always by a negative connotation, then its absence here comes as something of a surprise.

What this definition does do, however, is emphasise the specialised and purposeful nature of institutions. They are deliberately set up for particular reasons, rather than being organic developments which have broad and perhaps unspecified functions, such as a village or a town where people come together in a usually unplanned way to do many different things and for many different reasons. This element of deliberation and specialism is by definition 'unnatural', if natural is taken to mean unplanned and spontaneous, and perhaps in a culture which is suspicious of over-regulation and rationalism, this feels uncomfortable.

It is only when we come to the descriptive form of institution, 'institutional', that the negative connotations of institutionalism are referred to: 'dull, routine and uniform' is one of the definitions given alongside the example: institutional meals. When the dictionary comes to 'institutionalise', the evaluative element becomes even more apparent – the first definition given is 'to subject to the deleterious effects of confinement in an institution: a mental patient who was institutionalised into boredom and apathy'.

If the dictionary records are accepted as a reasonable account of how the words are used, then we can extract from this a variety of uses, ranging from the neutrally descriptive to the condemnatory. What the dictionary does not tell us, however, is how this move is made, how we have come to use institutional in such a negative way – it is not inherent in the idea of institution. 'Institutional' might just as well be used as a compliment, to denote places which are well organised and respected, but if it ever is used in this way, the dictionary does not record it.

From this discussion it is immediately apparent that the term institution cannot be taken for granted. We may use it as a shorthand for forms of care which we think are dehumanising and demeaning, but scrutinising these assumptions shows us that this shorthand is inadequate. Not only is it not necessarily accurate, because there are other things that the terms stand for, but it also limits our thinking. We find it difficult to escape the shorthand to think through these other things (the institution as a source of communal pride and achievement, or the institution as a manifestation of tradition and order), and these difficulties exist not only in our everyday use of the term, but also in academic use. In academic use, where it is often expected that terminology has undergone some rigorous process of checking, so that the terms are precise and unambiguous, the word institution seems to go unchallenged.

There are a range of settings which have been called institutions (hospitals, prisons, workhouses, etc.), with a correspondingly wide range of functions and features attributed to them (protection, segregation, therapy, punishment, etc.). In some ways this makes the term rather too broad to be useful. Conversely, the modern use of the term is quite narrow in its evaluative sense – calling something an institution is rarely complimentary and often derogatory and this narrowness also makes it difficult to use. Nevertheless, we have decided to hang on to the 'I' word because we feel that there is some value in the idea of using a word which everybody feels they can take for granted, and showing them that they cannot. The impact of this book is, we hope, that it will change ideas, and the best place to start in this process is from where people are at now. Starting off with taken-for-granted ideas seems to us a more open way of challenging them than either leading up to a challenge in a circuitous way, or simply ignoring them and, therefore, suggesting that they are not important.

At a pragmatic level, there is simply no other word that replaces the 'I' word. Instead of saying 'institution', we could use 'hospital, care home, therapeutic community, etc.', but this is cumbersome and will always run the risk of missing out some types of institution. In short, the 'I' word is useful as a general term for places in which people are cared for or receive services, and as a term which covers the 'family' of institutions that exists. The notion of a 'family relationship' type of definition is a useful one which has been most usefully expounded by the philosopher Wittgenstein (1958). He argued that we commonly use terms to cover a range of things, without expecting them to share defining features. The example Wittgenstein gave is of the term 'game', attached to many activities which upon examination have no single, shared, defining characteristic. They do not all involve competition or teams, some are amateur, some are professional, some are physical, some are sedentary. Wittgenstein pointed out, however, that we quite comfortably use the term despite this lack of precision, because what we see is a 'family relationship' between games. In a family, not everybody has identical features – some members have only the same colour hair, others only the same shaped nose –

but we can identify a family resemblance despite this variation in individual members.

We can use the term 'institution' in a similar way, to indicate a family of organisations which do not necessarily share a defining characteristic. They are not all coercive or punitive or therapeutic, or necessarily routinised or dehumanising, or healing, and they provide services for people with a range of needs (and not necessarily problems). This usage seems, to those who like their definitions to be precise, to be suspiciously woolly and likely to lead to vagueness and confusion. On the other hand, however, it frees us up to think beyond those defining characteristics that we have taken for granted in past debates, which have told us that our practice in institutions is doomed to dehumanise those who live and work in them.

The importance of thinking beyond these culturally imposed limits cannot be overemphasised if practice is to move forward. The next section in this chapter therefore provides an historical overview of the institution, in a range of guises and through different periods, in order to emphasise this point. As we look at the changes and developments in institutions, one thing emerges quite clearly – that the form of the institution is not inevitable, but is shaped by the society and culture in which it is created.

## Historical antecedents – an overview

Looking at language gives us some idea of the genesis of institutions, but the importance of looking at history is that it can let us see how things can change and develop, and it can serve to illustrate the extent to which external and internal dynamics come into play. This helps set current practice in the context of social and cultural mores, and gives some indication of what is possible and what is probable. In writing this book we were beset by the perpetual dilemma of boundary delineation: many of our exemplars so far derive from the fields of welfare (health, social care, social work) and we have also referenced educational and penal examples. These areas are central to our themes and we shall continue to build upon them. However, there are other relevant topics which will impinge (for example the provision of 'social housing'). Furthermore, the historical development of institutional living inevitably requires examination of aspects of social life which owe their origins to abandoned value bases and qualitatively differential conceptual analyses of society. For example, the Malthusian notion of 'laws of population' (1766–1834, published 1966), with its suggestion that the poor will always be present in society and that the problem is not amenable to management through social policy, is not a viable political doctrine today.

### SOCIAL FUNCTION OF INSTITUTIONS

Early institutions developed from the application of expertise and social influence to identified social need. People grouped together to share resources and knowledge. In this respect institutions for care made sense only when relevant expertise and knowledge developed (for example monastic orders and the growth of medical knowledge). Nonetheless, this model differentiates between providers and users of institutions, with all the nuances of language which we have already explored. Whilst monastic orders may have been rich and respected, the inmates (although some were rich and the purchasers of shelter) were, if objects of charity, not necessarily respected. In contrast, and in another timescale, the Quaker institutions such as the model villages at York (Rowntree's at New Earswick) and Birmingham (Cadbury's at Bourneville) attempted to treat people on rational grounds through a humanitarian approach to workforce management. The dilemma here becomes almost Foucauldian (Fox, 1993) in the sense of how far situations are defined by those who wield power: to what extent was the provision a means to an end rather than an end in its own right? It is arguable that philanthropy helped to create a stable workforce and that a stable workforce led to better levels of productivity. Here the very paradox of the notion of caritas becomes apparent, and it was these tensions which led, through a chronology of social progression, to the recipients of care themselves serving as mechanisms for the salvation of others, as witnessed by the 1834 Poor Law Amendment Act (referred to below).

## SOCIAL HISTORY

It will already be apparent that we firmly believe that the perspective of social history is crucial to the development of an understanding about institutions. However for those who have an interest in social history, as we have, there is always the danger of the historical becoming an end in its own right, and we wish to avoid such an imposition on this task. One of the key initial questions is to establish just where in history, and at what point chronologically, we should begin. The orthodox position is often to start with the 1834 Poor Law Amendment Act, since it was arguably this legislation which seems, from the perspective of some twentieth century writers, to have imbued the notion of state welfare institutions with a certain notoriety. It is tempting to point to the Boards of Guardians, Parish Unions and centralised Poor Law Commissioners as an emerging infrastructure for dealing with welfare issues, and indeed many social policy and social history texts do so (Forder's introduction to Hall, 1983). However, to collude unquestioningly with this notion would be firstly doing an injustice to much of the provision which existed at the time (McCord, 1979) but, more importantly, would also overlook the major achievements of social policy from the sixteenth to eighteenth centuries. We do not need to dwell on these achievements lengthily but, in the context of today's rapidly changing social policy and service delivery systems, we need as many indicators as we can find to help us recognise not only from where our institutions derive, but also what they might develop into. Much of the language which surrounds the Poor Law will, to the contemporary ear, now have a quaint ring of antiquity as well as an associated sense of redundancy about it. It is, nevertheless, illuminating to discover just how relevant many of these older concepts might be. Therefore, the selected identification of aspects of the old Poor Law era (that which predates the 1834 Act) is a useful anchor for developing a focused historical, social policy, economic and political perspective which continues to provide a current relevance.

The late Tudor approach to welfare, or poor relief (also known as the relief of distress) and the subsequent breakdown, towards the end of the eighteenth century, of systems enshrined in the 1601 revision of the 1597 Act for the Relief of the Poor, underpins any understanding of nineteenth century legislation. The institutions which were established during the sixteenth to eighteenth centuries formed the basis for development of the models for residential welfare settings of the nineteenth and twentieth centuries. Those historical origins and traditions still influence the impact of interdisciplinary boundaries amongst services which evolved from such widely disparate roots as the penal and health systems. And the historical issues of care versus control, containment versus treatment, and status versus stigma remain very much current and contentious issues. These are matters which are far from being consigned to the archives of social history and, indeed, are central aspects of institutions and institutionalisation which we shall address. By this we do not mean that such a position carries with it any implication that sixteenth century ideology and practice are inevitably relevant to our own society. Nor are we suggesting that contemporary society does not regularly encounter new and demanding circumstances which require new and imaginative solutions. However, it would be neglectful to ignore in its entirety the wealth of material which past experience has to offer, for every contemporary institution has an element of the historical enmeshed within it.

The central theme of the 1601 Act was the establishment of a national framework of locally administered and financed poor relief, and it was only when the population began to grow dramatically towards the end of the eighteenth century, bringing with it levels of distress which reached locally unmanageable dimensions, that the Tudor systems began to break down. These interesting tensions between local and national contexts are echoed in current social policy issues. An impossible burden was placed on the local rates, which had the secondary impact of keeping wages at an unrealistically depressed level, thereby threatening the very structure of law and order. During the intervening two centuries, however, the Elizabethan Act made important contributions to the development of institutional care. A famous quotation describes this as follows:

> The old poor law workhouse can be seen as the ancestor of most of the institutions which form part of the modern social services. They were used as old people's homes, occupational training centres, maternity, mental, and general hospitals, children's homes and hostels for the homeless. With their workshops, schools and sick wards they constituted the full range of welfare service in microcosm, from which the modern specialised institutions have grown.     (Oxley, 1974, p. 79)

Such an assertion might suggest an oversimplification of the case, since there are also numerous other aspects which contributed to the development of institutional provision. Nevertheless, Oxley provides a useful overview perspective. He was also writing at a time which predated the ensuing massive structural reorganisation of the welfare services. Paradoxically, the political thrust of government policy from the late 1980s was specifically designed to have the effect of recreating the notion of a unitary, or 'seamless', service.

One significant feature of the pre-1834 legislation was that it encouraged flexible responses to local need (Oxley, 1974), and there are examples of workhouses opening and closing in response to the vacillations of local harvest or trade cycles. The notion of out-relief, that is the provision of financial and material resources to impoverished parishioners, enabled families to survive hard times as a unit rather than be moved into the workhouse and lose their potential for self-help. However there are also examples which challenge an exclusively humanitarian interpretation of the prevailing ideology within the system (such as the workhouse test of the 1722 Poor Law Act, abolished 60 years later, which denied relief to those who would not enter the workhouse). The reason why the 1834 Act received such subsequent notoriety was that it abolished out-relief and introduced the doctrine of 'less-eligibility'. The latter meant that the circumstances of any person in the workhouse must be worse than those of the poorest person subsisting outside it. In other words, the Victorian notion of the 'deserving' and 'undeserving' poor was reinforced.

Essentially, though, it must be recognised that the role of the Poor Law was to complement and supplement the unmet areas of need between the vagrancy laws on the one hand and the charitable institutions on the other. Alongside the parish workhouse and penal systems existed philanthropic and religious charitable institutions which offered hospitals, almshouses, orphanages and schools. However, functions were not always necessarily discrete. The parish models drew heavily on experiences of the voluntary sector. Some quasi-penal settings were inherited by the parishes as part of their law and order remit.

The old Poor Law institutions defy easy categorisation, partly because the role of central government in this respect was permissive rather than directive and partly because of the lack of sufficient reliable and meaningful data. It is, however, clear that there was considerable variety in the range and quality of service provision (see McCord, 1979 for examples).

## ORIGINS OF INSTITUTIONAL WELFARE SERVICES

In the post-1834 period there was a burgeoning of legislation and service development which reflected the enormous demographic, social, economic and industrial changes which took place in the Victorian period. Within this social context there was an exponential growth in the development and pro-liferation of institutions. However, there is little to be found by way of a trad-ition of truly generic literature in tracing their history. In 1777 John Howard's seminal work, *The State of the Prisons in England and Wales*, led to a review of the conditions and purposes of the penal establishments, and was directly responsible for the introduction of innovative and relatively less harsh regimes for young offenders (including the development of Parkhurst Prison on the Isle of Wight as a model institution for wayward boys). These regimes in turn led to the establishment of Reformatory and Industrial Schools – first piloted in Scotland – which were later reclassified as Approved Schools by the 1933 Children and Young Person's Act, and subsequently incorporated within the Community Homes structure introduced by the 1969 Children and Young Person's Act. The background to these and other services specifically provided for children and young people is well chronicled (see, for example, Stewart and Tutt, 1987). Contemporary accounts survive from the mid-nineteenth century (e.g. Carpenter, 1851 in Manton, 1976) and there does exist a comprehensive literature which records, updates and analyses events up until the present time (e.g. Cadbury, 1938; Burlingham and Freud, 1944; Aichorn, 1951; Heywood, 1965; Carlebach, 1970; Berridge, 1985; Rose, 1997). Similarly there are developments which emanated from the introduction of the national education service and Bridgeland (1971) explored the historical background and major issues relating to the special school movement for children deemed, at that time, to be classified as maladjusted. In a more general way the seminal work of Pinchbeck and Hewitt (1973) explored the position of children (and, by its very nature, makes reference to the experiences of adults) in English society from Tudor times until the mid-twentieth century. This impressive piece of work contains many contemporary accounts of institutional life for children throughout the ages, including a graphic description of the living circumstances of child labour in the mills.

Perhaps the most comprehensive generic literature in existence is that which is a product of the poor law institutions referred to earlier in this section. Whilst the pre-1834 legislation enabled the provision of locally determined services for the meeting of local conditions and needs, the 1834 Act abolished out-relief (except for sick and aged paupers) and ensured the introduction and maintenance of a nationwide network of permanent parish institutions. Cowie (1973) developed a reference dictionary of British social history which is a useful guide to identifying the relationships between the various institutions, both in terms of chronology and function. And the classic nineteenth century texts of Mayhew (reprinted in 1967), *London Labour and the London Poor*, provide fascinating insights into the lives of the poor of London, particularly of 'those that will not work'.

In a similar vein, the literature relating to mental illness covers the 'lunatick asylums'. Scull (1979, 1981; also in Tomlinson and Carrier, 1996) has written at length on the historical developments, whilst Goffman's challenge to the internal perceptions of a large American state mental hospital will be considered in some detail in the next chapter. The history of the institutional treatment of mental illness, together with that of learning and physical disabilities, is dispersed amongst the various records and writings on asylums, colonies, hospitals and pauper institutions.

Included in any inventory of relevant literature must also be the descriptions of the activities of the charitable and religious institutions. Baglee's (1971) study of a charity hospital is but one example of a hospital which was, in essence, a home for older people rather than a place for medical treatment in the modern understanding of the word. Thus, whilst it is clear that there exists a great deal of literature concerning the welfare oriented institutional services, historically there does not exist a unifying perspective which can bring together the components in a coherent, integrated way.

It is also clear that there are a number of themes which emerge from a study of the poor law era which are, at least in some respects, recognisable as significant factors which impinge on practice today. Major topics include the 'relief of distress', the 'care versus control' debate, and the associated issue of dependency versus independency. Equally significant are the economic and political perspectives.

Furthermore, we need to acknowledge the fundamental question of whether or not the notion of the relief of distress (social, personal, physical or material) is tenable today. The evidence from studies concerned with assessment of client needs tends to support the view that state funded health and welfare agencies continue to operate on the basis of confining their activities to the relief of distress, in the sense that their scope is defined through statute and they are not empowered to expand their functions beyond such a remit. It is increasingly apparent today (Tester, 1996; Nocon and Qureshi, 1996) that as the demand for services increases in response to demographic development, the assessment process is used as much to exclude from service delivery as it is to include. However the nature of the statutory framework which informs practice is itself informed by a far wider range of perspectives than was the case in earlier times. In particular, professional opinions and public pressure exert a considerable influence: for example, the politico-economic thrust of the Thatcher years led to the closure of large-scale long-stay institutions, a move which has now been questioned as a result of high profile tragedies, which have identified the failure of community care policies and strengthened professional concerns.

Similarly the notion of whether or not individuals and categories of people merit intervention from public funds remains very much a live issue. The concept of the 'deserving' and 'undeserving' poor may be easily recognised through the distorted lens of history, resonating with Mary Carpenter's nineteenth century description of vulnerable children as 'perishing' or 'dangerous' (with the former in need of help, and society being in need of protection from the latter). Whilst Carpenter was a champion of causes for children in need, she clearly found no contradiction in her attitudes. Such a view is not far removed from some more recent attitudes in relation to criminal justice and mental health care and the associated tensions between prison, hospital, residential hostel and care in the community. Interestingly the language was also reflected in a text by Hoghughi (1978) entitled *Troubled and Troublesome*, which explored issues relating to children and young people.

One feature which, as we have already seen, occurs consistently in any writings to do with institutional care is that of dependency. Indeed, to many the function of any institution will create dependency. However there is substantial contrast between public belief and expectations, and the reality of much effective residential living. We acknowledge today that institutional care which creates dependency can lead to higher mortality rates in older people; that concepts of rehabilitation are as important as retribution and public safety, though all must be tempered with a concern for the safety of both the individual and society. More significantly, the notion of independency needs has been addressed in considered, evidence-based practice and theory. Examples include the work of therapeutic communities such as Peper Harow and the Henderson Hospital, and the writings of Davies Jones (in Courtioux *et al.*, 1981) as well as others previously cited.

Finally, for this chapter, are the economic and political contexts of change. The economic factor is an important one, especially in determining levels of service provision and development, for any welfare system can only spend according to its national wealth. Historically the nation could, through either public or private wealth, afford the great gothic buildings of public and philanthropic welfare; today it cannot. Residential care is a service industry which is essentially labour intensive. The drain on social security and health resources which contributed substantially to the development towards care in the community for older people, away from residential nursing and social care, was equally influential in the residential child care sector. Annual returns of the Chartered Institute of Public Finance and Accountancy (1975) show that historically 50% of the revenue budget expenditure of social services departments in the 1970s was allocated to residential services. This figure has since been in steady and dramatic decline. When in competition nationally and locally for scarce resources, residential care is often deemed to be too expensive; and when it becomes necessary to look for economies within a budget then it is often relatively more feasible, in both organisational and operational terms, to close a unit than to seek alternative and more complex remedies. There is often a tendency to argue that non-institutional alternatives will be both cheaper and better, even though the evidence may not necessarily be produced.

Inevitably linked to the economic factor, though separate from it, is the influence of local and national political perspectives. Perhaps of most concern within the context of this book is a consideration of the relative merits of the statutory and independent sectors (the latter including charitable, not-for-profit and commercial sectors). There is a compelling argument which suggests that it is morally unsatisfactory for all social and welfare responsibilities to be delegated to public officials and institutions, for at some point individual and community accountability and responsibility become lost. Successive Conservative administrations from 1979 to 1997 offered incentives to the independent sector to extend their areas of operation in direct relationship to the decline in the activities of the statutory services residential provision. The private sector growth of residential services for older people, the increasing transfer of funding from institutional to community based services, and the closure of the long-stay geriatric, psychiatric and mental subnormality hospitals, as they were then known, are all examples of efforts to reduce long-term state managed care services and to divert the responsibility for funding and capital investment to the private and voluntary sectors (as well as to service-users). Evidence presented to the Audit Commission (1985, 1986) demonstrated an accompanying shortfall of planning and funding in many instances, and this position was reinforced by the Griffiths Report (1988) on the realities of implementing community care-based policies.

What this material demonstrates is the way in which the context for change in residential services is an historical one which introduces new dimensions to existing perspectives as society develops. Rarely is there ever a clean break with past models, and rarely do models continue to exist for long in unchanged form. However a point does come where the cumulative emphatic influence of change does lead to an essentially differently evolving service. We seem to be at such a point now, though it is not a position which is precisely or narrowly defined in temporal terms. What this change seems to imply, at least in some senses, is that we need more clearly than ever to understand where we have travelled from, and where we might aspire to reach. Tomlinson and Carrier (1996) remind us of 'Scull's dilemma' with its suggestion of institutional neglect being superseded by community neglect and the consequent implication that there must be an alternative to both. Our view is very firmly that there is a place for institutional care, and that it can be an effective and preferred mode of practice.

Overall there exists no powerful, unifying tradition of history within the professional practice of institutional care, and no consensus of what are the key issues and watersheds. It is, however, our contention that within a pluralistic service delivery system in health and social care, residential care has much to offer, and that it is possible to point to a developing conceptual framework upon which to base our position. The function of this discussion is to enable us to contextualise our exploration of what precisely institutional care has to offer its users, and how best to develop good standards of professional practice. In particular, we wish to present a book which has an applied focus for residential practitioners in social and health care. We hope that this will reflect the developing interdisciplinary activity between the two sectors and bridge the changing boundaries of *ad hoc* initiatives. In doing so we hope to develop a model of evidence-based practice and theory, a model which will contribute towards the integration of the hitherto often discrete practice and languages of health and personal social services into a coherent and integrated social and health care approach.

# 2 Current research and policy debates: implications for practice

Introduction

Policy/academic literature

Pro- and anti-institutionalist positions

People who are in institutions

Practice in institutions

## Introduction

With such an unintegrated pedigree the development of an integrated overview of institutional welfare services might seem a rather daunting prospect. Whereas formerly the services were able to exist in a degree of isolation from one another, it is now becoming increasingly necessary to have some means of conceptualising a changing and ever more complex and sophisticated model of welfare. This process has been under way for some time, though our concern now is to look back over the past 30–40 years or so. There are a number of significant components, both of process and context.

To try to understand these we have to go beyond everyday language and dictionary definitions to examine some of the information which has shaped ideas about institutions – in other words the body of writing and thinking which has gone on in academic and professional circles. These discussions, of course, carry great weight and authority because of the expertise and rigor which we assume is brought to bear in these circles. The impact of these debates, then, is not just a reflection of the level or quality of analysis that they involve, but the confidence that we have in their conclusions. As ideas move from research through the media into everyday talk, then, the processes of checking and criticism are sometimes bypassed. It is sometimes very important to take received wisdom and subject it to critical scrutiny.

# Policy/academic literature

The academic literature on institutions is, of course, vast, and we can do no more than sample it. It is more pertinent in the context of this book to try to identify some common themes and patterns, because this work is not a collection of individual researchers and writers working in splendid isolation, but a representation of the efforts of a community of academics who reflect and reference and respond to each other. In the work on institutions it is possible to trace the development of ideas as they are proposed, adopted and modified through time. This notion of tracing does tend to oversimplify the process of academic debate and makes it seem more rational and systematic. It is, nevertheless, an instructive process as we can identify what have been seen as key figures in the field, and how their words of wisdom have been incorporated, sometimes uncritically or unknowingly, into the work of those who have followed.

## GOFFMAN THE DEMOLITION EXPERT

Jones and Fowles (1984), in their overview of research on institutions and institutionalism, cite a number of texts which, they argue, set the parameters for all work which followed them. One of the texts, which they describe as part of the 'springs of protest' against the institution as it had developed in this century, is that by Goffman, published in 1961, entitled *Asylums: Essays on the Social Situation of Mental Patients and Other Inmates*. In the preface to this book, Goffman states that his belief is 'that any group of persons – prisoners, primitives, pilots or patients – develop a life of their own that becomes meaningful, reasonable, and normal once you get close to it . . .'. What Goffman produced was a description of the lives of groups of people in what he calls 'total institutions', which does indeed seem to get close to and make these lives intelligible to the reader. What Goffman describes is a life in which the inmates' every activity was totally regulated by the institution, where their meals, their recreation, their daily routine, were all governed by the institutional routines – hence the term 'total institution'. Goffman describes this reduction in autonomy and choice as a process of dehumanisation which results in a loss of a sense of personal identity for the inmates.

   Goffman details the way in which this happens, the processes and practices which make up 'institutionalisation', and chronicles the minutiae of life in these places, and the ideas and motives which underpin the form it takes. He discusses ideas about containment and control, about depersonalisation and stigma, about inmates as people with 'spoiled identities', people who are no longer regarded as competent and normal members of the human race, but who are discredited as unable to make choices or decisions. Similarly, the staff of these institutions become somehow less than people in their formal role of custodian, which constrains and shapes their actions too. Indeed, Goffman's account, while in one way a vivid account of life in institutions, in another way reduces our sense of the people who live and work in them as being people like us – Goffman's description reduces them to shadowy, symbolic figures. We hear none of their words or accounts of their experiences directly; this is filtered through Goffman's eyes and voice.

Jones and Fowles describe Goffman as a 'radical' among the 'demolition experts' that they identify. This term suggests, however, a degree of commitment to change which is not necessarily apparent in Goffman's work itself. The concern seems to be to describe, in sociological terms, a particularly interesting cultural phenomenon; to forge an agenda for change was not Goffman's purpose. The attack on the institution comes from some abstract realm of theory rather than from the experiences of those who have been part of an institution, and it is the theoretical audience that seems to be the main target, rather than those in practice or policy makers. Nevertheless, the work of Goffman is valuable in the way it challenged the orthodox view that institutions were a necessary evil in society, simply by the degree of description that he provided about the minutiae of daily life in them. It is quite possible that until this work was published, those who had thought about institutions had not really known much about how they operated, or how the broad framework of services was translated into practice.

## FOUCAULT AND DECONSTRUCTION

Foucault (1965) provides another example of a theoretical approach in the analysis of institutions which forms part of his work. As one of those writers generally termed 'post-modernist', his general aim was to challenge the notion of 'progressive development' beloved by those who believed that the modern world, with its assumed more rational and effective structures, represented an improvement on what had gone before. What Foucault and his colleagues argue is that there was no such progressive development, and what history demonstrated was that ideas and practices simply changed, often in a disconnected way, and that the views of one era were not superior to any other – they were just different. The notion of institutions as rational and enlightened solutions to social problems was therefore suspect, and the anomalies of this view were to be made evident by a historical analysis of thought and ideas – an 'archaeology of knowledge'. The methodology of this was the deconstruction of ideas and debates. Rather than taking documents and records as straightforward statements of fact, they were viewed as documents shaped by the dominant ideologies and power structures of the time.

In this archaeology Foucault writes of the institution and the way he takes it to be an instrument of social control and symbolic of the attempts of rationalists to impose order on the human condition. His thesis draws upon historical material, but the 'histoire' that he presents in respect of institutional care is one which has been challenged on grounds of accuracy and interpretation (Jones and Fowles, 1984). Nevertheless the argument that part of what institutions do is to bring under surveillance areas of life that were once private and personal, and that they do so under the auspices of rational arguments about scientific solutions to social problems, is one which is hard to discount entirely.

Perhaps the most serious problem with Foucault is his notion of 'judgmental relativity', that no judgement is necessarily better than another, that because knowledge is a creation of power and influence there is no certain and enduring knowledge. This puts us in a difficult position as practitioners or policy makers. If institutions were simply an exercise in power rather than a scientific or rational move to address the problems or needs of society, as was confidently assumed at the time, then our suspicion of rational thought in the past also has to extend to any rational or scientific recommendations that we are making now. If we suggest, on the basis of current research, that institutions should be changed, or even closed down, we are on no surer ground than any other society in the past. They too thought that they had the most valid knowledge and the most sensible approach, but according to Foucault they only reflected the power structures of their time.

The deconstruction of institutions, then, also seems to provide few indications for moving on, or at least suggests that if we do move on we are not necessarily going anywhere better. In the meantime, however, there are hospitals, residential homes and other institutions with clients and staff in them, who, we strongly suspect (after Goffman) are not enjoying a therapeutic or constructive regime. This gap between the theory of Foucault and the experiences of practitioners and clients has been summarised by Porter (1996) when he discusses the potential impact of the Foucauldian analysis on nursing:

> In many ways the exclusively critical nature of Foucauldian thought has not mattered too much up until now, in that his influence has been largely confined to non-vocational disciplines such as sociology and philosophy, whose ruminations have little direct effect on the outside world. However, its import is far different when it starts to influence practical health care disciplines such as nursing. While critical deconstruction of existing nursing practices is undoubtedly beneficial, it is not enough. Nurses need to identify more effective forms of action and interaction. At this point Foucault can provide little guidance. (p. 227)

Again, like Goffman, Foucault's concern is not to provide a programme for practice development, but to alert us to the problems in what we are doing now. In taking us thus far along this line of thought but no further, however, these authors seem to be sending us a pessimistic message, holding out no hope for change or indications as to how it might be achieved. Goffman does not address the question of why the institutions developed in the way that they did and Foucault, even although he chronicles change, does not attempt to explain how it happens – both writers describe institutions as if they were inevitable and beyond the power of practitioners to change.

## SZASZ – A FREE-MARKET VIEW

Another demolisher of the idea of institutions as solutions to social problems is Thomas Szasz (1961) who has a practitioner background as a psychoanalyst. His argument, to simplify a huge body of work, is that we are mistaken about the social problem that mental hospitals are supposed to address. He disputes the idea of mental illness, arguing that another, more valid term for this behaviour would be something along the lines of 'problems of living' and that our response to it, particularly the institutional response, is demeaning and robs people of their liberty and rights. By calling behaviour mental illness, we take away responsibility for this behaviour and, by placing people in institutions, we perpetuate this irresponsibility. We take away opportunities for people to control and manage their lives – the institution does it for them.

Szasz, therefore, portrays the mental hospital as an infringement of civil rights and an invitation to abandon all sense of personal responsibility, a portrayal that fits in with some aspects of other analyses of institutional care. Szasz, however, goes further than simple demolition, but suggests alternative solutions to the behaviour usually termed mental illness. First, it should not be described or excused in such a way, but should be subject to the same legal and criminal justice rules of all other behaviour. This tension between the defence of civil rights and the seemingly paradoxical adoption of a criminal definition of some of the behaviour of those who are termed mentally ill, is, at the very least, interesting. It alerts us to the notion that if we choose to think of people who are mentally ill as being responsible for their actions, thus avoiding the demeaning view of them as not responsible (as, for example, we view children) then the corollary of this is that we make them subject to the same forms of social control as everyone else. Szasz's second assertion is that where therapy is desired by individuals, it should be contractual therapy, i.e. privately funded therapy in which the client is a willing partner who is paying the bills and calling the shots. Where people without the money to pay for these services fit into this system, however, is not very clear. The alternatives, therefore, raise a lot of questions – moving from collective and state-organised provision to individual and personally funded therapy is not a panacea. While Szasz's analysis, like those of Goffman and Foucault, sensitises us to the ways in which we can identify problems with institutions, his practitioner background does not necessarily make for anything other than limited and problematic alternative strategies.

## PERPETUATION OF IDEAS

Demolishing institutions then, seems to have become a popular activity in academic circles. As Jones and Fowles describe it, the academic literature has often been 'uncritically rejected by practitioners, who found them unhelpful, and uncritically accepted by academics and their students, who have turned such concepts such as "total institution", "institutional neurosis" and "carceral power" into catch-phrases' (1984, p. 1). Such a dichotomy serves, perhaps, as a sharp reminder of the power which can be exerted by the institution.

The acceptance and perpetuation of such catch-phrases is problematic for several reasons. Firstly if these ideas form the assumptions on which research is based, then all research does is perpetuate these assumptions by seeing research data through this lens. The research question becomes, 'what form is institutionalisation taking here?' rather than, 'does institutionalisation exist?' or, 'is this the best way to describe what happens in an institution?'. If ideas of institutionalisation become so embedded in the researcher's mind that they are not critically examined but simply taken for granted or not even noticed, then we cannot expect research to produce much that is challenging to these ideas. What results is 'academic stereotyping', in other words that teachers and researchers start to think in the rigid, simplistic and unchallenged ways that they are so keen to point out in other people.

Baldwin *et al.* (1993) illustrate this process when reviewing some of the literature in the area of residential care for older people. They begin with Townsend's (1962) study, evocatively titled *The Last Refuge*, which authoritatively describes such care in a way which invites or suggests no other possible interpretations:

> In the institution people live communally, with a minimum of privacy, yet their relationships with each other are slender. Many subsist in a kind of defensive shell of isolation . . . they are subtly orientated towards the system in which they submit to orderly routine, lack creative occupation and cannot exercise much self-determination . . . the result for the individual seems fairly often to be a gradual process of depersonalisation. (p. 79)

Baldwin *et al.* argue that Townsend's work resonates through much of the research which has followed, leading to researchers isolating the institutions from the wider social context in which it exists, and from the personal lives and experiences of the people who live in them. The research, therefore, concentrates on the dynamics within residential homes and not on the wider social and personal processes at play. The authors give examples from some of the research in the 1980s which has had this focus and which, moreover, starts from the assumption that residential homes share the characteristics of Goffman's 'total institutions', and that these institutions exercise a uniform and inevitable debilitating power on residents.

They cite, for example, Wilkins and Hughes' (1987) evocation of the concept of 'total institutions' in their description of the process whereby older people surrender to 'enforced dependence in the institution' and give other examples of influential research which has started off from the same point. They argue, however, that 'It is no longer helpful to assume that there is one institutionalisation process which in all essential respects is unaffected by culture, the economic context, the service organisation in which the residential establishment is located and so on' (p. 74). They also identify aspects of Goffman's work which has been neglected, namely the 'inmate world' of which he gives a detailed account. The idea of residents actively negotiating their residence and the ways in which they cope with or resist the institution seems to have been bypassed by Townsend's depiction of their passivity.

Baldwin *et al.*'s (1993) analysis of the power of academic stereotypes of institutions not only shows how these stereotypes shape research, so that researchers effectively predetermine the way in which they will collect and analyse data, but it also identifies another way in which uncritical acceptance of the idea of the damaging institution can influence debates and ideas. They point to the corresponding evaluation of community care projects for older people, where, they assert:

The net effect has been for the 'worst' features of residential care uncovered by the researchers to be contrasted with the 'best' features of community care. By default, the influential institutionalisation studies of the 1980's lend weight to an uncritical view of the superiority of care in the community which may not be borne out by the reality.

(Wilkins and Hughes, 1987, p. 75)

Ideas about institutions, then, can shape not only our evaluation of this type of care, but also of the alternatives. We may not just be uncritically hostile to institutions, but uncritically approving of anything else.

Approval for alternatives to the institution was also supported by research and literature which concerned itself with 'dysfunction'. Much of the literature of the 1950s–1970s, with negative messages for institutions, had a fundamental and dramatic impact on institutional care and collectively became known as the 'literature of dysfunction'. The early attachment theory work of Bowlby (1953) promoted the supremacy of the maternal relationship and was critical of family-alternative child care regimes. Ivan Illich (1971) was extensively critical of the developing state macro-institutions of the twentieth century. The work of Goffman (1961), again, and Polsky (1962) investigated the negative and damaging effect of some forms of institutional provision. In particular, large psychiatric hospitals and reformatory institutions have frequently evoked concern in terms of both their internal practices and their public images. However the post-Second World War culture, with its new welfare state provision and specific commitment to exorcise what was popularly viewed as the spectre of the poor laws, reacted with some fervour to these criticisms of its services.

The detail of the 'literature of dysfunction' has been analysed elsewhere (Stanley, 1978, 1989; Walton and Elliott, 1980; Jones and Fowles, 1984; Jack, 1998) and is not accepted uncritically. Its overall impact was to challenge the basic purposes and achievements of institutional care as well as to add to the body of available knowledge. Some of the effects were rapid and overt, for example the post-Bowlby development of 'family group homes', which focused on the 'housemother' as a surrogate parent and the closure of some of the very large institutions. Others were of a more indirect nature, for example the promotion of specialised foster care for adolescents as a replacement for residential care. However, the very real difficulties of managing the individual and community problems of the most damaged, disturbed or vulnerable people were undervalued. Care workers in many settings found their functions undermined and their purposes ill-understood. The significance of this material cannot be underestimated, since it is popularly blamed for the poor image of many institutions and their workers. However, that is an inadequate and partial view: the negative aspects which were identified undoubtedly existed and required to be remedied. More importantly, this literature tended to rely overly on the individual case study of a narrow and highly specialised nature, and became extended improperly to a generalised application.

## POWER OF ACADEMIA

The academic discussion of institutions is important because of the power and influence which academia enjoys in society. While we may be disparaging about the 'ivory tower' , nonetheless those who are thought of as living there are also thought of as being intellectually able and learned. It is, therefore, difficult for those outside this world to develop any coherent challenge to this debate which might go beyond dismissing it all categorically as esoteric nonsense.

The academic view of the institution, therefore, carries a weight which extends to other forms of discussion and discourse. At the same time, the traffic is not simply one way. Everyday talk does not just simply mimic the talk of the academics and, indeed, it is arguable that academic talk must come from or begin with the talk that everyone else uses, since academics are, after all, members of the human race. Nor is it simply the case that everyday talk is simply a sloppy version of academic talk, where concepts are misinterpreted and used uncritically, for we have seen that this can happen in the academic world too. Perhaps it is, therefore, safest to say that whatever uncritical use of words is evident in everyday talk, it is given some sense of validity and respectability by a similar use in research and teaching. Without any check on this process of mutual validation, and without any attempts to challenge stereotypical thinking, we can all happily continue to use the language of institutionalisation, secure in the belief that this use has been confirmed by research.

## POSITIVE PICTURES

Interestingly, at about the same time as a body of literature was growing up which depicted institutional life as dehumanising and dysfunctional, another set of accounts was developing which suggested that this was not inevitable and, indeed, that life in institutions could be of positive benefit. Initially there were the highly personalised, often idiosyncratic accounts of practitioners who wrote both to record their own experiences and to promote their own methods and philosophies of care and treatment: Richard Balbernie (1966) and David Wills (1971) in the field of therapeutic communities for disturbed children, A.S. Neill (1970) in liberal residential education, Maxwell Jones (1973) in therapeutic communities in the mental health setting. There are many more examples. The strength of such writing was that it contributed to a developing knowledge base, complementing – but not always engaging with – developments in the social sciences. Much of it, in contrast with the moral and penal reform motivation of the nineteenth century developments, leaned heavily on a psychodynamic orientation and the maintenance of a medical model of treatment. It also enlisted a following of support which promoted adherence to such approaches.

A significant difficulty in terms of the wider development of services was that the leading practitioners, almost without exception, were character- istically charismatic personalities upon whose individuality and flair the success of their methods and establishments depended. It was also characteristic of such leadership that their management styles were essentially autocratic, even when the residential community model was founded on a form of democratic partnership. Such a style demonstrated many of the traits of a closed, pioneering service. In spite of the effective work which was able to be undertaken, there was little likelihood of the records giving as high a profile to the failures of the system as it did to its successes, and those successes were scarcely likely to have been recorded in the most objective of ways. Perhaps the single unifying characteristic of such practitioners was their tolerance and understanding of those for whom little tolerance existed elsewhere in society.

## DEVELOPMENT OF AN INTEGRATING CONCEPTUAL FRAMEWORK

There is also a 'composite' literature which has explored the positive perspectives of institutional living. There is no evidence that this has been an orchestrated movement, but rather a piecemeal development of independent perspectives which are capable of collective appraisal. Perhaps one of the most significant texts in this respect is that by Wolins (1974).

Wolins is important for two major reasons. First, along with others, he was responsible for coining the use of the term 'group care' as a generic term which might embrace a wide range of diverse activities. This term, which has generally failed to gain universal currency, has been explored at greater length by Ainsworth and Fulcher (1981). Second, he drew attention to the positive applications of institutional care and living which could be found. The very title of his book, *Successful Group Care*, echoed his thesis. He argued persuasively that there was abundant evidence to suggest that not only were there many alternative models to the natural family for the nurturing of children, but also that these alternative models were able to raise children whose activities and aspirations were socially acceptable rather than aberrant. He further explored some of the literature of dysfunction, demonstrating some of its weaknesses, demonstrating an impressive capacity to reframe the critical positions and offer alternative interpretations.

This theme was further developed in *Revitalizing Residential Settings* (Wolins and Wozner, 1982). This text was aimed at the 'caretakers' in residential settings and its purpose was to argue that institutions are a necessary part of contemporary society, and also that their regimes were seriously flawed and in need of improvement. This was an important key text but unfortunately its complex arguments and somewhat tortuous prose militated against it having any profound impact in the UK.

## Pro- and anti-institutionalist positions

In recent years then, the research verdict on institutional care has been mixed. The exposés of institutional care had aroused concerns about standards and practices, yet at the same time some forms of group care and group living seemed to be having some success. The positions adopted by people on the two sides, the pro-institutional and the anti-institutional, took various forms, but the debate seemed to focus on a number of key tensions. The first and most obvious tension was between the idea that care and support could and should be collectively structured, as in therapeutic communities, and the opposing view that it should be provided on an individual level. The collective/individual debate is, of course, usually one of ideology primarily and only secondarily one of empirical evidence, and it comes with a lot of associated ideas and disputes. To simplify the positions, the collectivists tend to see the human condition as essentially a social one, with interaction and mutual responsibility between people as being the basic currency of the way in which we live. This view tends to portray people as essentially benign and supportive to each other, and motivated to work for the common good. Individualists, on the other hand, see the human condition as an individual one, with each person having unique characteristics and needs. The individualist point of view is suspicious of notions of 'fraternity' amongst people and concentrates on the rights of individuals to protect their own interests in the face of competition or interference from others.

The collectivist/individualist positions are evident in other tensions in debates about institutions. The debate about freedom, for example, is construed differently depending on which side of the debate is talking. Collectivists might not emphasise individual freedom as much as the collective good, or might see the institution as being a haven of freedom in a repressive society, the case with such insitutions as Peper Harow (Rose, 1997) and Summerhill (Neill, 1970). Individualists, on the other hand, may regard the very fact of being in an institution as being a restriction of liberty, even if voluntarily entered into. The implications of having to modify conduct in order to fit in with the wishes of others are disconcerting to contemplate, and daily life in institutions necessarily involves an erosion and invasion of personal domains which is an anathema to individualists. Moreover, the experience of being in an institution can be damaging to future freedom – the notion that institutionalisation saps the will and encourages dependency.

## POLICY DEBATES AND DEVELOPMENTS

These tensions are also played out in political debates, as policy is developed around the core values of the groups in power. Policy decisions are not necessarily a matter of judiciously considering empirical evidence – they shape and are shaped by the political and cultural climate of the times. Hence in a number of government reports (see Chapter 3) we find that one of the baseline assumptions that they display (either explicitly or implicitly) is that the case against institutions is taken as proved. This discourse, however, takes place in an environment in which Western governments, particularly in the USA and the UK, were beginning to articulate more strongly the virtues of independence and freedom, and indeed to campaign on the platform of reducing state intervention in the lives of the populace.

To this debate might also be added the variety of official investigative enquiries which have been conducted in and around the field of institutional care. One of the more significant relatively recent examples of which has been the Wagner Report of 1988, set up to review the

> role of residential care and the range of services given in statutory, voluntary and private residential establishments within the personal social services . . . to consider . . . what changes, if any, are required to enable the residential care sector to respond effectively to changing social needs. (p. 1)

The report itself was disappointingly brief and its recommendations bordered, at times, on the simplistic. It is arguable that the brief was too wide to enable a substantive enquiry to be undertaken. Furthermore, its committee sat at a time when the shape of its focal services was destined to undergo extensive future change with the introduction of the National Health Service and Community Care Act of 1990. Accompanying the Wagner Report was a more substantive volume entitled *The Research Reviewed* which, whilst commendable for the breadth of user groups embraced, was also unsatisfactory since it focused unduly on historical issues which have been chronicled often enough (we are in danger of repeating the offence ourselves!) and thus failed to take advantage of an important opportunity to contribute to the more complex matters of contemporary development. A chapter on 'common issues' singularly avoids any discussion in depth on a definition of residential care:

> . . . no definition has been agreed, but at the minimum, residential care involves the provision of both accommodation and care on the same site. (p. 42)

An independent national enquiry, initiated by the Secretary of State, ought to have been capable of a more considered debate than this extract indicates. Furthermore the sections which dealt with the individual user groups do not seem to take into account the available generic work which might have been used to inform their writings. Atkinson's bland assertions that:

> Residential care, in relation to people with mental handicap, has a short history. It may have a restricted future . . . . Residential care evolved from institutional care . . . . (p. 127)

are characteristic of a disingenuous approach which fails to achieve an integrating theme. Paradoxically, the cumulative impact of the literature survey leans towards a negative interpretation of residential care, in contradiction to the approach declared by the report's title, *Residential Care: A Positive Choice*.

In 1967 the Williams Report, initiated by the National Council of Social Service, surveyed demand, conditions of work and the nature of the residential task in over seven thousand 'Old People's Homes, Children's Homes, Other Homes, Special and Approved Schools, and remand Homes' which accommodated between them some quarter of a million people. Whilst outcomes were substantively concerned with staffing, the report contributed for the first time a general picture of the residential care field.

The discrepancies of style and achievement between Williams and Wagner serve perhaps to underscore the increasing complexities of institutional health and social care. In 1967 it was possible to produce a convincing, if incomplete, study which looked towards the future in a constructive and positive manner. Over two decades later an exercise with similar associations was able to combine only a poorly integrated overview with expressions of blandishment and concerns. Wagner, having spawned an influential working party, continues to stand today as a major reference point for social care, despite its shortcomings.

## RECENT ANTI-INSTITUTIONAL POLICY

Despite the limitations of official reports, such as the Wagner Report, an anti-institutionalist stance is implicit in recent policy documents in the UK, particularly the debates leading up to the National Health Service and Community Care Act of 1990. The White Paper which preceded this, *Caring for People* (Department of Health, 1989), for example, sets out the aims of policy as being to provide the services and support which people need 'to be able to live as independently as possible in their own homes, or in "homely" settings in the community' (1.1. p. 3). Implicit in this statement is the assumption that the best place for people to receive care is in 'the community' or at 'home'. Policy equates this with personal choice, independence, and 'normal life'. Corresponding developments in shorter hospital stays, and the increase in day care treatment, also rely on the implicit support of the idea that institutions are bad places to be, and that no-one really wants to be in them unless it is absolutely necessary. The case that care in the community is inevitably a preferable alternative to institutional care has been challenged vigorously by Scull (in Tomlinson and Carrier, 1996), who recognised the operation of institutional forces in the community

Cynics may argue that these policy developments are a result of fiscal, rather than ideological imperatives, in other words that the move to community care is an excuse for cost cutting and reduction of services. This may be the case, and it is certainly an accusation that has been levelled at governments, but it is interesting to note that this accusation is presented as a claim that policy is not 'really' in favour of community care, or is only paying 'lip service' to the idea. There are very few who publicly questioned the fundamental notion that community care is a better alternative to care in institutions.

More recently, of course, as stories have hit the headlines about people being discharged too early and unwell from hospital, or people with mental health problems posing a threat to others, more criticism of the idea that community care is desirable and appropriate for everyone has been voiced. In the case of people who are viewed as receiving inadequate or truncated treatment, the complaint is often about cost cutting, but in the case of people with mental health problems, the disquiet is more complex. Public fears about safety lead to calls to keep 'dangerous people' off the streets, a position which betrays little concern for these people's welfare, but action groups, such as

MIND, make the argument that some form of institutional care is the most appropriate place to receive some forms of treatment. Their concern with the welfare of those who need care can, disquietingly, sound very similar to the views expressed by those who are concerned with 'public safety'.

The subtleties of the arguments are not best served by the way in which they are sometimes conducted. Pressure groups, politicians and the media can, in a 'sound-bite' culture, rely heavily on graphic and shocking images of neglect and suffering, whether caused by people being in institutions or by people not being in institutions. Throughout these debates the 'institution' is often implicitly defined by its alternatives, for example institution as opposed to 'home' or institution as opposed to 'community'. Again these terms are used in a shorthand way, but a further problem of the discourse here is that it is circular. Home is what is not an institution, and an institution is what is not home. The community is not an institution, and an institution is not a community. However, such reasoning is scarcely sustainable in either logic or practice.

## THE IDEA OF 'HOME'

It is worthwhile trying to unpack these contrasts a little further. What, for example, is a home? The dictionary definition is surprisingly unhelpful at first glance – the first meaning given is simply 'the place or a place where one lives'. Later definitions, however, are more illuminating – to feel 'at home' is to feel 'at ease'; if something is 'close to home' then it is 'concerning one deeply'. We have then a sense of a place which is not simply somewhere to live and carry out daily functions, but a place that is comfortable, familiar and, moreover, somewhere to which there is some sort of attachment and link with personal identity. Dictionary definitions, however, only take us so far – they reflect the common usage of a word (as far as the compiler is aware of it), but do so in a way which can sometimes only raise further questions: what for example is meant by 'at ease' or 'deep attachment'? These ideas have been explored further, however, by researchers in the social sciences, and their comments certainly suggest the complexity of what it is we mean when we use the word 'home'.

Sixsmith (1986), for example, comments on the range of definitions available in academic literature, concluding that, 'Unfortunately [they] tend to present a set of rather disparate ideas and observations' (p. 281). These ideas have included the home as a 'social unit' created through kinship ties and the home as a vehicle for self-expression and identity, in other words a site of cultural activity and also individual identity. This paradox between definitions which are based on notions of cultural participation and, simultaneously, individual preferences, suggest that 'home' is a place with many dimensions. As Forrest (1983) has argued, the home is something which says something about us as individuals.

Following this idea we can see that our ideas of our selves and our homes are intimately connected; it then follows that for each individual self there is a different set of characteristics which he or she takes to be definitive of 'home'. In Sixsmith's phenomenological study these ideas were 'suspended' while data were collected and participants asked to participate in a multi-sorting task. The results of this suggested that many conventional uses of the term 'home' have been oversimplified. For example people can have more than one place which they call home, and that a place can change its status – places can cease to be a home, or grow to be one, depending on a wide range of personal circumstances.

Amidst these shifting sands, it is also important to point out that it is somewhat simplistic to equate home with happiness; in other words some homes are places where people can have damaging or unpleasant experiences, although Sixsmith's data suggest that in these circumstances they might cease to be described as home. These personal debates, however, are not always echoed in official definitions of home as simply being the place where somebody lives.

The complexity of definitions of home goes some way to suggest that using this term as a self-evident contrast to the institution is fraught with problems. This is not only because home is a personal and perhaps unique construct, but also because none of the qualities or characteristics is necessarily or automatically excluded from what happens in an institution. An institution does not *necessarily* prevent the development of self-image or the expression of personal identity, and it may have cultural and social dimensions to it. Some institutions, however, do seem to foster particular self-images and cultures which we do not feel are desirable or healthy, but it is important to point out that there is nothing inherent in the institution which produces this effect. There are a number of examples of religious and academic institutions, and indeed institutions which provide health and social care, which facilitate identities largely regarded as positive. Thus we can argue that an institution may become home, in a range of ways, to those who live in it.

## THE IDEA OF 'COMMUNITY'

Similar problems occur when we look at the other antithesis of the institution – the community. Again the dictionary definition is starkly phrased: a community is (1) the people living in one locality and (2) the locality in which they live, but again this is later elaborated on by reference to common characteristics or interests. The two dimensions of community are, therefore, place and people but, as with so many dictionary definitions, this is perhaps an oversimplification.

Cohen (1989), for example, has argued that a community is defined by boundaries which are largely symbolic, in other words that their establishment rests on agreed ideas about who is 'in' and who is 'out'. As such, then, they depend as much on exclusion as on inclusion. This argument also suggests that notions of locality as being the main dimension of community may have to be modified and, indeed, the way we talk about communities suggests that we have no problems in thinking of a locality as housing a number of different communities. Any big city, for example, is likely to contain a number of different religious, ethnic, or cultural communities. Furthermore, the development of symbolic rather than concrete boundaries suggests that people can feel that they belong to a community which does not necessarily have a distinct geographical base.

Notions of community invoked in debates about care seem to carry implicit assumptions of homogeneity in localities, that a community can be defined simply by geographical dimensions. Locality may be important in a person's way of defining their own community, as it may be in the way that they define their home (and the two concepts can be indistinguishable at times), but it is not the only factor. This observation calls into question simple geographical ideas of community, and also raises some questions about ideas of delivering care in this way. For someone to be part of a community, and supported and accepted and cared for by it, or within it, requires more than them simply living there. Their place in relation to symbolic boundaries must be such that they are within these. Thus someone can physically live in a locality, but not be part of a community.

## People who are in institutions

Our discussion of the concepts of 'home' and 'community' have shown that they are ambiguously defined and used, and we have indicated that some of the things that they represent or stand for are not necessarily excluded from institutions. Perhaps the negative image of institutions is related to the purposes with which they are credited. Prisons, for example, are institutions which incarcerate and punish and indeed some of us would be very disappointed if they do not do this – witness the furore over reports that prisoners are enjoying themselves in any way. Similarly, mental hospitals are seen as places of control and coercion, again something that we might approve of (for the protection of others) or feel to be necessary, but nevertheless lead us to feel rather uneasy. These institutions may be performing what we feel is a useful function for society, but it is a necessary evil with which we are not entirely comfortable.

On the other hand, there are some institutions that have purposes with which we are comfortable. The general hospital which provides care and treatment for the sick, for example, can and has been constructed as a benevolent institution. Institutions which give shelter and care to the needy, hostels for the homeless or homes for abused children, for example, are also institutions which it is possible to think of as having laudable aims. Between the extremes of benevolence and containment there are, of course, many variations and ambiguities, where institutions have multiple goals and aims, some of which may seem paradoxical. Interestingly, it is possible to identify these paradoxes by distinguishing the way some aims are about development and support of those who live in the institution, while others are about their restriction or even punishment.

The purposes of an institution are, of course, linked to the way that those who live there are regarded in society, and it is difficult to distinguish between the stigma attached to the people in the institution and that attached to the institution itself. When we look unfavourably on certain groups, such as prisoners, people with mental health problems, or drug addicts, then the place that houses them becomes disparaged. Conversely, we look on some groups with sympathy and understanding, such as those who are ill (through no fault of their own, of course – people who are seen to court illness are a different matter), or children, who are largely seen as innocent victims unless, of course, they have committed a crime, in which case they become a menace to society. Their institutions can be portrayed as havens of care and support.

Regardless of the benevolence or otherwise of the institution, however, spending some time there seems to distinguish some people from others. Having been brought up in a children's home, for example, is held to be a salient and distinguishing characteristic of people, no matter how much or what they have done since this. We read reports of court proceedings, where defendants are described as having been 'in care', and this information is produced as some kind of explanation for the defendants' behaviour, either as a defence or almost as another accusation. For those who have achieved success in later life, being brought up in a children's home is also viewed as an integral part of that person's identity, and also as an explanation for behaviour. A children's home can be a spur to achievement in the way that it stimulates children to escape both it and the whole world of welfare.

What seems to be going on here is a form of 'second-order institution-alisation' where identities are 'spoiled', to use Goffman's term, in an inevitable and irrevocable way. The circular logic goes something like this: institutions house people who are not normal, who need support or supervision in ways that normal people don't. You are, or have been, in an institution, therefore you cannot be normal. Hence people who live in institutions are regarded as institutionalised by definition, rather than because of any evidence that we have about their behaviour. Older people in residential homes, for example, can be dismissed as confused and dependent, simply because we presume that that is why they are there, and these dismissive assumptions can prevent us from seeing and respecting any evidence to the contrary (Reed and Payton, 1996). We tend to reify the institution, to endow it with almost invincible power to crush those who live there, and so all behaviour is interpreted as evidence of institutionalisation. If older persons in residential care say that they like living there, this is interpreted as evidence of an institutionalisation process which has robbed them of their critical faculties. If they say that they do not like living there, then this is interpreted as a maintenance of critical faculties despite institutionalisation.

Among the plethora of voices, those who condemn institutions and those who support them, some voices and experiences seem, therefore, to be lost. Critically, these voices belong to those who spend more time than anyone else in institutions: the clients and the staff. Much of the debate assumes that the clients can be 'spoken for', in other words that the words of researchers, politicians, and civil servants can effectively represent their experiences. There is, however, some research which seeks to do this more directly, by focusing on the clients' experiences and views and eliciting first-hand accounts of these. This category of literature comprises the narrative, autobiographical, biographical, and even fictional accounts which derive from the experiences of institutional care services, together with an increasingly influential element which reflects the consumer's perspectives, written by the consumer. Tizard, Sinclair and Clarke (1975) wrote a significant text on the varieties of experience of residential care. Writers such as Lasson (1981) and Whittaker (in Clough, 1988) have reported on research studies of consumers' views. Ethnographic accounts of life in residential homes for older people, such as those by Gubrium (1975, 1993) have the potential to change our views of residents as passive and inactive, and to reveal a social world which is dynamic and in which participation is skilled and thoughtful.

## Practice in institutions

Another element which can be connected to the way we think about institutions is what we know, or think that we know, about what sort of activities take place there. From the press there are occasionally appalling reports about cruelty and deprivation which provoke debates and concerns. Sometimes these are met by or coincide with official responses which involve inquiries and court cases, which in turn receive wide publicity. Popular fiction and drama show us, in dramatically convincing ways, how people are treated by callous or sadistic staff.

In addition, as discussed earlier, there are a range of academic reports and studies which have investigated life in a range of institutions. These studies have tended to portray staff as being victims of the institution as much as the clients, or as being deprived of opportunities to develop and change. Menzies (1960), for example, in a discussion of ritualised and depersonalising nursing practice in hospitals, suggested that the reasons for the fragmentation of patient care arose from the inherent anxieties in working with people who were suffering. Organising work through depersonalising rituals was a defence mechanism against this anxiety – the only way of coping that nurses had been able to develop in an organisation which did not recognise the nature of their work and was concerned to deny or suppress their problems. Similarly, Miller and Gwynne (1972) described two models which staff adopted in the care that they gave: the 'horticultural' and the 'warehousing' models, which they had developed in the face of any other apparent alternatives.

This is the more sympathetic portrayal of staff – the other view is that they are people without compassion or integrity, who are lacking in motivation or ability. Much of the research about staff attitudes fits into this category, as researchers describe 'bad' or 'negative' attitudes and link these to malpractice. While such research often suggests training packages as a 'cure' for these attitudes, the analysis does not often go beyond this to consider the wider social context in which people practice. In addition, much as the residents of institutions are portrayed in the literature, staff are described by researchers, rather than describing themselves. One vivid exception to this format is the book called *Keepers: Inside Stories from Total Institutions* (Glouberman, 1990), which contains transcripts of interviews with people who work in a range of institutions. While this book does allow staff to present themselves to the reader, however, it is by no means the case that there is no filtering mechanism – the very title, in its dramatic evocation of repressive regimes, creates a negative framework in which to place the content.

In contrast to these images, there are others which portray what goes on in some institutions as therapeutic and beneficial, and staff as benevolent and caring. Ideas about some institutions include stories about vocational impulses which transcend privation or discipline and which somehow lead to personal growth and development. Films about visionary founders of movements and institutions such as children's homes emphasise the shelter, care and succour that is found there and which was created by these charismatic leaders. Dramas based in institutions such as hospitals or universities stress the collegiate nature of the relationships between the people there, the sense of belonging that they have, and the support that they give the institution. As recruitment strategies, these may work very well with naïve youngsters, but these fictional narratives are not found in the research literature on staff in institutions, and the commitment of staff is only paid lip service by politicians as they close down services or introduce cuts in provision.

Staff, therefore, seem to be subject to a process of second-order institutionalisation similar to the process that clients experience. Because we have vivid images of some authoritarian figures who work in institutions (such as Nurse Ratchet in the film *One Flew over the Cuckoo's Nest*), this influences the way we view other staff. To work in an institution is, therefore, to behave in the way that the institution imposes, to dehumanise clients and to behave unthinkingly or sadistically. With little literature to challenge these images, apart from the charismatic rebel of fiction representing the exception which proves the rule, those people who do work in institutions are offered little in the way of positive images or courses of action to take.

Some ways of developing practice are, however, offered by some research which has attempted to represent and address the interests and needs of those who practise within the settings. This research was aimed at assisting those who worked within institutions to make more sense of their working environments and to produce findings which could help conceptualise and improve practice. This material was important because it would contribute to the development of a knowledge base with a greater degree of practice application, and also assist in the development of institutional care as a method of working in its own right. This latter is what Courtioux *et al.* (1981) describe as 'living with others as a profession'. Examples here include the work of the Dartington research team into residential environments (e.g. Millham *et al.*, 1975), many research projects undertaken under the auspices of the ESRC Children in Care Programme (Clough, 1988), and the theoretical work of Ainsworth and Fulcher (1981) and Fulcher and Ainsworth (1985) in developing the notion of group living.

This work is vitally important for developing practice in institutional settings, and will form the foundation for much of the rest of this book. We end these first chapters, then, with a positive note after the negative and sometimes depressing material we have covered in this section. We have moved from a consideration of lay language and its negative portrayal of institutions through to an historical overview which showed that institutions are diverse in terms of their purpose, their ethos, and the way in which they are regarded by the rest of society. We should also acknowledge the collective power, for good or for ill, of the institution. Summarising the research literature has shown that the rigor that we assume accompanies the process of academic debate is not necessarily, or always, evident, and that academic work can perpetuate as well as challenge stereotypes. The relationship between research and policy is often tenuous, with ideology often determining which research is valued and which is not; which ideas are accepted and built into the foundations of policy, and which are rejected and dismissed.

# Identifying the issues    3

If it is important to establish that the major professional purpose of working and living within a care-oriented institutional context is to facilitate the quality of the lived experience or the development and maintenance potential of interpersonal exchanges, then it is equally important to establish the focus for such input. We have already demonstrated that there is a wide range of models of institutions, and that whether or not institutions are valued is in part dependent upon how their function is perceived within society. However, there also exists the crucial question of how the institutions are perceived and experienced from within. In this chapter, we are not so much concerned with revisiting the conceptualisation of institutional characteristics as looking at some particular examples, identifying the detail of the perceptions and developing a taxonomy of enabling and disabling functions. Perhaps it is closer to the spirit of our approach to reframe this objective: we shall consider firstly the positive functions of enabling institutions, and then look at how some functions can disable institutional care, leading the latter to be experienced as a disabling organisation.

## Fundamental paradox

We should perhaps also keep two further thoughts at the forefront of our minds as we explore this material. In the first instance it is unlikely to be the case that any welfare-oriented institution established within our society will adopt objectives which set out explicitly to damage service-users. Even though there are numerous examples – from the Staffordshire pin-down enquiry (Staffordshire County Council, 1991), where a method of physical restraint was identified as abusive, to nurses who have been convicted of killing their patients – these are instances of where the informal systems have largely been allowed to develop unchecked by the formal. However, these examples also serve to remind us, secondly, of the inevitable number of examples which are cited about bad, or damaging, care experiences. This paradox lies at the heart of all institutional care: how is it possible to achieve a high quality lived experience *and* to avoid unacceptable, damaging practice?

We firmly believe that this paradox can be addressed usefully, even if it may be not easily resolved, but that it requires an empowering of residents on a scale with which not all care settings might be able to cope. It is axiomatic that relationships, the building blocks of living together, can and do break down. It is, therefore, imperative that within the institutional environment there are systems which do not just accommodate, but proactively manage, such breakdowns; we shall develop this theme further. One key to making progress is to acknowledge the importance of appropriate sharing of functions between staff and residents. However, for now we are more interested in pragmatically establishing functions which can help us to identify and assess standards of practice in the first instance.

Quite often when groups are asked to produce an inventory of positive and negative functions of group living – try it out for yourself, using your own rather than others' experiences – the results can be contradictory. In other words, what some might judge to be a positive indicator will be viewed by others as negative and possibly, though not necessarily, vice versa. For instance, 'house-rules' which might be introduced for the benefit of the majority may be seen as punitive by the minority. We should not be unduly surprised by this, since individuals will arrive at their own conclusions from differing life experiences. However, such a phenomenon does serve to give some indication as to why it can prove so difficult to establish living regimes which are able to satisfy all users. Not only must all systems learn to accommodate all users, all users must learn to accommodate all systems and it is precisely this dynamic process which should be focal to all institutional environments or, as Moos (1974, 1987) described them, social climates. Below we have clustered some of the positive and negative functions, translatable into best and worst practice, which have been generated from some of our own classroom activities in working with both pre- and post-qualifying students, at non-graduate, undergraduate and post-graduate levels, in nursing and social work. Having identified them, we shall then explore them further within the context of concrete examples from practice. For the purposes of this chapter we are concerned more with the nature of the material covered in the accounts of practice and the nature of their outcomes, rather than rigorously presenting an inventory of conclusions, though some of the latter do, of course, feature.

## Best practice – functions of enabling institutions

Maslow's (1970) hierarchy of human needs has yet to be bettered in offering a model through which to introduce the essential elements of the lived environment. Whilst it may be possible to level accusations against it of being hackneyed and ageing, it continues to provide an unsurpassed and authoritative rubric: for it is impossible to deny the sheer versatility of its basic simplicity. However, Maslow can only really provide a framework for exploration and analysis and cannot, in spite of his apparent omnipresence, address the heart of that with which we are centrally concerned – how to implement and sustain best practice standards. We can learn from Maslow how to shape the 'what', but not so clearly the 'how' of effectively managing the institutional regime. Thus, we can recite what we already knew: that to cater for basic human survival needs is a prerequisite for the successful development of higher order activity. Psychotherapeutic interventions are not of the highest priority if the stomach is empty. Unless it is possible to deliver the raw essentials of food, warmth and shelter, we cannot begin to make progress with the 'higher order' activities of self-actualisation and social harmony. For even at this very, very simple level of debate the complexities can appear daunting.

The graphic accounts by Rose (1997) of issues surrounding the provision of food and shelter at Peper Harow (see below), demonstrate only too clearly how and why the institutional provider is faced with such a substantial challenge. If we are partly defined by what we eat, we are also equally partly defined by how we provide food for others, and our values systems become translated into public statements in so doing. We shall explore this issue in greater length in due course. For the time being, however, we would simply want to express the importance of providing properly for the 'lower order' needs, whilst not wishing to understate the difficulties that this will create.

Maslow's seductiveness is that he provides such an appealing and all-embracing model that it sometimes seems as though there is no need to look further. It must, after all, be self-evident that we all share common values in terms of how we would wish to treat others. It is relatively simple to develop a list of all that should exist. An enabling institution will also offer health and social care, and provide a context for the development of interpersonal relationships and group support. It will offer solace and peace of mind. Self-empowerment can be achieved through enabling attitudes and advocacy strategies. It can engender self-help and access to resources and information. A sense of community and belonging can enable physical and emotional development. It can be experienced as safe, but can also be a means of maintaining functional contact with the 'outside' world. It can offer a means of interrupting a dysfunctional cycle of behaviour or experience. Put quite simply, there is ample evidence to support a view that the institution can be a place of choice, a better place to live than that experienced previously: an asylum in the truest meaning of the word. Perhaps all of this can best be summarised by suggesting that an effective institution can accommodate the individual and community needs for dependency, independency and interdependency.

However, it is not possible to point to a text and say with confidence, 'here is an example of good or bad practice', without first addressing the range of issues outlined in Chapter 2. Who is writing? Why is it being written? What is the style of content: how subjective or objective is it? What is the conceptual foundation? These are not easy questions to answer. When judgements are made they have to be based upon some kind of evaluation. If a study is aimed at trying to tease out how to develop, describe or evaluate practice, then at least there is a hopeful basis for expecting to find useful indicators for best practice. Even so, the reader can often be left with an impression that the poor practice is to be found in the evidence and that the good perhaps exists only in the aspiration.

One example of such a text is Clough's *Old Age Homes* (1981). This is a fascinating account of a research study conducted essentially through qualitative methodology which included participant observation and the administration of various interviews and life satisfaction tests. In spite of the passage of time since its publication – some of the language is outmoded and Clough acknowledges that notions of consumerism are only just becoming major issues – the study raises issues which would be recognised by readers today. The myths and paradoxes of homes for older people, the golden years of later life versus the evils of institutionalism, activity versus inactivity, engagement versus disengagement, dependency versus independency, are all to be found. There is much descriptive detail and plenty of hypothesising. Nevertheless, however accurate and detailed a picture the study might offer, it does not lead to a clear enunciation of positive practices and experiences, and the examples appear to be overwhelmingly of poor, or not good enough, practice. Thus in a study which is both insightful and compassionate, and which was undertaken to give pointers to the development of good practice, there is little by way of positive evidence from practice to assist the reader in developing their own.

## EXAMPLES OF POSITIVE PRACTICE

In our work with students the following issues have been identified by them as key positive functions of institutional care:

- Meeting basic human needs: food, clothing, shelter, health care, personal safety.
- Meeting social needs: companionship, group support, supporting routines (practical and emotional), structure, controls, protection for self, protection from others.
- Meeting emotional needs: sense of identity, sense of self-worth, sense of belonging, peace of mind, alleviation of pressures.
- Meeting personal needs: access to resources and information, ready availability of attention, wider choice, a focal point from which to develop, a means of interrupting a dysfunctional (for whatever reason) lifestyle, a better place to live than before, mechanisms to enable appropriate dependency, independency and interdependency needs to be met.

These headings and their contents are neither exclusive nor exhaustive, and the verbs which qualify them are diverse: to provide, enable, facilitate, tolerate, condone, and so on. The headings are not unique; there are many inventories of need, Maslow's being a case in point. Furthermore, there are also a number of inventories of principles of care which cover very similar areas. For example, *A Better Home Life* (Care Centre for Policy on Ageing, 1996) identified issues such as fulfilment, dignity, autonomy, individuality, esteem, quality of experience, meeting of emotional needs, risk and choice: a list which is almost exactly analogous, though articulated in different terms.

What is significant about the students' list is that it is a distillation of issues raised by practitioners in pre- and post-qualification and registration learning. These are characteristics which those who undertake to care for others believe are important.

Relatively few recent studies exist which explicitly search out examples of best practice and then offer any kind of substantive analysis. Below, we identify a number of quite different examples, using as a framework the functions listed above, together with a number of questions which we have already identified.

## Rose (1997)

Entitled *Transforming Hate to Love*, this book is an outcomes study of the treatment process at Peper Harow, a residential setting for adolescents. Rose had written previously (1990) of his work as director of this former approved school turned therapeutic community. Set up in 1983, leaning heavily as a basis on Erikson's (1959) model of psychosocial development, and operating within a psycho-therapeutic framework, Peper Harow worked with the most demanding, rejecting and rejected of young people. Rose left in 1983 and the institution closed in 1993. So this is a post-experience exploration, but one which consults those who went through the process.

There is no shortage of good practice guidance in this study; from the imperative that however troubled or resistant the young persons, they were not admitted unless they volunteered to attend, to the assertion that the personal qualities of staff were their greatest resource. This is essentially a narrative which derives from Rose's personal vision, but the story is related with conviction and relies for its authentication and persuasion upon the voices of the young people who experienced Peper Harow. Most importantly, it is based upon detailed personal evidence set within a potentially replicable regime, though that is not to underestimate the levels of difficulty experienced by Peper Harow in sustaining its approach. Rose does not attempt to hide the disasters and tribulations, for it is also his contention that their task was an ongoing one where success was not measured episodically but over time, and in the full awareness of the range of experiences and behaviour to which a community is witness.

In summary, Rose differentiates between the type of daily regime in the old approved school and that of the therapeutic community, arguing that change cannot be achieved by simple imposition of will. He contrasts learning mastery of a skill as an end in its own right with the individual's development of self-management skills through the medium of activities. Rose acknowledges that it is notoriously difficult to compare outcomes between different types of intervention. However, he also asserts that the chief agents for change were a combination of a variety of experiences within a psychotherapeutically oriented, appropriately resourced, environment which pays careful attention to detail. The practitioner can turn to this text and learn from positive examples which embrace the entire life-space of the institution as a vehicle for personal growth and development.

## Burton (1993)

In *The Handbook of Residential Care*, Burton presents a practical guide for the institutional worker. It is based upon his own experience of living and working within institutional care, and is related with enthusiasm and a concern for passing on his conviction that care homes can offer positive and rewarding lifestyles. The focus of this text is to explore, within a context of direct personal work, the role of staff in the institutional setting. Its approach is essentially experiential and pragmatic and, like the Rose text, there is ample illustration from staff and user perspective alike.

Of particular interest in Chapter 8 is a series of interview vignettes, which demonstrate a wide range of user perspectives on their experiences and which reinforce the view that rarely is any experience ever all bad or all good. The final chapter echoes a theme which is close to our hearts in the conceptualisation and rationale for writing this book. It is entitled 'Liberating institutions' and closes with the words:

> I believe that existing institutions require collective vision and commitment, creativity and cunning, militancy and energy (some of the qualities we bring to direct work with people) to transform them from centres of oppression into places of liberation and life. It can be done. (p. 185)

This book is significant for the sheer quantity and detail of its material. It is grounded in a theoretical approach to professional practice, based upon extensively recorded personal experiences, and incorporates a substantial reference to a relevant literature. Perhaps most importantly, however, it is based upon providing accessible and usable material for the practitioner to incorporate into his or her practice.

## Reed and Payton (1996)

*Working to Create Continuity: Older People Managing the Move to the Care Home Setting* is a research report of a project which was funded through a Department of Health post-doctoral fellowship and the authors are academics with nursing backgrounds. The study also differs from the previous two above in that there is an emphasis on tracing a transitional process. Presented as an orthodox research report, it offers an overview of the literature, a detailed reporting on research methodology, findings from the data on both decision-making and early days in the care home, as well as offering findings which consider the longer-term processes of adjusting to life in the care home setting.

A particular feature of the research was an overarching concern to discover the individual perceptions of older people involved in the process of moving into care homes, together with some of the interviews providing follow-up perspectives a year or so after moving. This report captures a widely varying range of experiences and responses. The authors identified that much of the literature reviewed had an anti-institutional stance, and the study aimed to:

re-examine this view by shifting the focus from the scientific and quantitative lens of objectivity and measurement to the more subjective and qualitative lens of story telling and narrative, seen largely from the older person's point of view. (p. 23)

The rationale for taking this approach is given as a response to the developing demand for consumer and user perspectives. Contrary to the views characterised in the 'literature of dysfunction', the study found that:

residents are frequently active and interested in the community dynamics of the home in a way that challenges the stereotypical images of passivity in these 'homes'. (p. 81)

Here, then, we have a study which challenges the prevailing orthodoxes and concludes that residents' relationships with each other are fundamental to their daily social experiences. These conclusions are, arguably, enabled by a research perspective which refuses to collude with the dysfunctional theories of institutional social and health care and which, to the contrary, maintains that the degree to which residents work at adapting to their new environments in positive, functional ways remains largely unacknowledged in the literature.

## Mallinson (1995)

Finally, in this trawl of positive exemplars, we consider *Keyworking in Social Care*. Mallinson is a social work educator with a long-standing interest in social care and particularly in keyworking, the subject of his PhD thesis. This text was developed in partnership with the Social Care Association/British Association of Social Workers and differs from the previous texts considered in this section in that it is a largely theoretical work. However, the material is grounded in practice examples and its primary purpose is one of practice development: there are very few sources of this nature to which the institutional worker can turn. It is written from a stance which is predicated upon the utility of institutional care. Its major weakness is a structural one: with no index there is a certain difficulty in using it as a reference source, even though the table of contents is relatively quite detailed. This is a great pity for a potentially important text.

Mallinson examines the origins of keyworking in group living, drawing an analogy with the case work process of field work whilst acknowledging certain fundamental differences, for example the multifaceted aspects of the keyworking role within a group context. The underpinning theoretical perspective is based upon a systemic approach and he draws on models and examples from a range of different service user groups: settings for older people, special education, day services, domiciliary services and residential child care. One major aspect which develops earlier, relatively simplistic, notions of keyworking is the linkage which is made between individualisation and the group. Mallinson proposes a structured approach which embraces care planning, individualised care, team working and management, each of which is examined in considerable detail. It is not our purpose here to do anything other than identify key issues, but this is a text which rewards careful consideration and offers a real opportunity to examine theory-based practice in a detailed, reflexive way.

## Worst practice – functions of disabling institutions

With the availability of such positive influences how, then, can it arise that so much of the reported evidence is of negative, disabling experiences? How, with the dedication of significant levels of resource, can institutional 'care' so often be characterised by such appalling standards that it is difficult not to share the outrage of the banner headlines? Perhaps part of the answer is that a considerable number of people who enter the care services as a profession are ill-equipped to survive the hothouse environment, and some are simply damaged and damaging adults themselves, as was acknowledged by the report *Children in the Public Care* (Utting, 1991). Another part of the explanation is that the damage experienced by service-users is sometimes so great that they themselves have learned, above all, to hate rather than love, and that the systems which should exist to provide safety and support become bureaucratised and insensitive. Selfishness, vulnerability and greed become inextricably mixed with fear and an uncritical quest for self-survival. The differentials between standards of private and public behaviour go unchallenged and unexamined. As a result, systems and working practices can become distorted and lead to disempowerment and oppression. The potential for abuse increases with the creeping growth of petty bureaucracy and the creation of cultures of dependency. Loss of individuality is experienced by service-users and staff alike. Concepts of dignity, privacy and individuality become first dulled and then disappear almost entirely.

In a context where the marginal or unacceptable behaviour becomes commonplace it can very quickly become mainstream and acceptable. As Institutionalisation (with a capital I) takes hold, the environment becomes more inward-looking and creates mechanisms which increasingly hold the outside world at arm's length. There is reduced contact with relatives, friends and independent perspectives. Individuals suffer from the negative effects of institutional stigmatisation, and become 'lost' in the system. Quite basic needs become neglected. Negative role models flourish and the negative power of the peer group, as first noted by Polsky (1962), rules supreme. Power and control is exercised through regimes of oppression. At another level it might simply be that staff do not possess the necessary skills to sustain a positive culture. Individuals lose all confidence in the capacity of the institution to change.

This is a depressing picture to paint, but it would be naïve and dangerous to pretend that it is not a realistic one. We shall explore examples of such institutional breakdown and endeavour to learn some lessons from them. Whilst it might feel better by far to try to learn from good practice, it would be simplistic to imagine that there are not good reasons to try to understand, and to learn from, the worst of practice.

## EXAMPLES OF WORST PRACTICE

In our work with students the following issues have been identified by them as key negative experiences within institutional care:

- Personal – self: loss of individuality, loss of self-confidence, loss of identity, loss of dignity, loss of independence, loss of choice, potential to become lost in the system, restriction of personal liberties, dependency, oppression, disempowerment, lack of privacy, enforced conformity, isolation, powerlessness, basic but not social needs met.
- Personal – family: family guilt, rejection, loss of contact.
- Structural: rules, potential for abuse, petty bureaucracy, stigmatisation, dumping ground/abandonment, cost or lack of resources, lack of trained staff, rigid regimes, lack of guidelines, lack of accountability, hostility from local community, quality of care variable – a lottery, easy option for dealing with social problems, hierarchy/authority of staff.
- Staff world: poor working conditions, low self-esteem of staff.

This is a devastatingly powerful inventory. Whilst the categories into which we have chosen to sort the items are inevitably open to interpretation and rearrangement, they nevertheless point to a problem of inarguable dimensions. Unlike the positive list earlier, the issues themselves cannot safely be presented as a matter for interpretation. Neither can it necessarily be said of them that their mirror images might be seen as the opposite, i.e. positive, as could sometimes be the case of the positive-attributes inventory. The list recognises that the problems are both personal and structural, but we should note that the language which is used to define the personal negatives is unremitting in its stark identification of the unacceptable. These data merely echo in overview the content of the literature of dysfunction, but in so doing serve to remind us that this is no distant, academic exercise, but rather that we are listening to the voices of those who are in close contact with service delivery. These are informed statements which we cannot afford to ignore.

Unlike the previous section, there exists no shortage of studies which actively search out examples of worst practice. Because of this, we have chosen to present two 'collections' of reports which represent two very different types of publication. The first is taken from a section (3.4) on inquiry reports in Kahan's (1994) *Growing Up in Groups*. This is a somewhat idiosyncratically presented text which presents an enormously detailed case for the implementation of more standardised principles of good practice; however, it does not offer any substantive discussion or analysis of the issues raised. It is packed with information and declarations of good practice guidance though, with no index and the bibliography presented in an unconventional format, its content is relatively inaccessible as a reference source. The second is Warhaugh and Wilding's chapter 'Towards an explanation of the corruption of care' in Allott and Robb (1998). This latter is one of six chapters which comprise section 4, entitled 'When care goes wrong', of a book which is presented as an introductory reader in health and social care. The section explores at some length examples of abuse in the care system and the chapter which we examine here is an abridged version of a paper which was published initially in the journal *Critical Social Policy*.

## Kahan (1994)

Kahan (1994, pp. 45–54) very briefly and selectively overviews eleven different reports covering the years from 1988 to 1993. These reports range over subjects which are variously broad and specifically focused. Included as examples of the broad approach are the Wagner Report (1988) *Residential Care: A Positive Choice*, where the material which Kahan focuses on serves once more to highlight the discrepancy between the content and the title, and the Utting Report (1991) *Children in the Public Care*. This latter was a government review of 'all matters bearing upon residential care' (Utting, 1991, p. 3) and which made thoughtful and well-argued recommendations in relation to the role and functions of institutional care, the welfare of children, management and resources. Both of these reports place a significant emphasis on the negative experiences of institutional care before presenting inventories for change. Examples of the specifically focused approach are the 1992 Ty Mawr Community Home Inquiry, which investigated this Welsh home following incidents of self-inflicted injury and suicide amongst residents. The inquiry was strongly critical of major facets of the regime and its management, recommending that the home should close. A further example referred to by Kahan was the Leicestershire inquiry of 1993, which investigated long-standing abuse of children by a care worker and highlighted detailed failures of management in Leicestershire Social Services Department that extended over a considerable period of time. This report was less concerned with making recommendations for practice than establishing culpability and systems failure. These specific reports serve to remind us, if reminder is necessary, of the unremitting catalogue of disastrous events which are to be found when care goes wrong.

Taken collectively, the reports are usefully presented as expressions of general concern at the quality of institutional care and government responses to those concerns. What Kahan sets out to do is to present the evidence and synthesise from it what she calls an 'essential message' (p. 53). In doing so the material is subjected to a level of reductionism which renders it almost bland and which is not subjected to any effective level of analysis. Furthermore, the basic paradox remains unaddressed: that there is an eloquently argued case for the use of such services, set in the context of examples of their catastrophic breakdown.

## Wardhaugh and Wilding (1998)

The second 'collection' of reports, the paper by Wardhaugh and Wilding (in Allott and Robb, 1998, pp. 212–29), is presented in a very different manner. It is essentially a scholarly analysis of a very wide range of institutional failure across the health and social care spectrum of provision. Its effect, in terms of institutional analysis, is as a latter-day Goffman. Through the extensive citing of sources the authors develop an inventory of eight propositions upon which to base an analysis of 'corruption of care'. These propositions are that corruption of care:

- depends upon the neutralisation of normal moral concerns;
- is closely connected with the balance of power and powerlessness in organisations;
- is associated with particular pressure and particular kinds of work;
- is underlaid by management failure;
- is more likely in enclosed, inward-looking organisations;
- is characterised by the absence of clear lines and mechanisms of accountability;
- can be induced by particular models of work and organisation;
- is encouraged by the nature of certain client groups.

Whilst it is beyond the scope of our purposes to undertake a detailed commentary on this material, there is a great deal of reasoned analysis within the text. It is important to establish what it is that the authors are attempting to achieve. Unlike the previous examples in Kahan's work, which focused on desired outcomes, Wardhaugh and Wilding are concerned with the detailed analysis of events and their associated contexts in order to discover the pre-conditions which must be met to satisfy the condition which they describe as the 'corruption of care'. Their work does not aim for an outcome in terms of developing good practice, but it does serve to further reinforce our understandings of institutional breakdown and, in their own words, their propositions 'are not all relevant in all situations but they are certainly helpful in pinpointing circumstances in which care systems are at risk' (p. 228).

One implication of this approach would be to develop a diagnostic tool which can be used to test for institutional health and its potential success or failure in broad terms. Overall, the material which we have reviewed in this section forms an important part of our thinking about worst care practice. However, in view of the fact that neither the types of examples nor their unacceptable outcomes are newly discovered in the history of institutional care, it is clearly arguable that there continues to be a missing component, a component which might help to ensure the pervasive development and maintenance of good practice. We shall explore what this component might look like in due course.

## What does all this mean?

It can seem self-evident that these issues are often no more than different facets of the same dilemma. Facets which are clearly and positively articulated in the best practice examples, but which become terribly confused in worst practice situations. Readers who are familiar with nursing and care systems will be only too familiar with the opportunities for personal development which arise around the provision of such basic commodities as food and clothing. How is it purchased? Who exercises choice? Who wears/eats what? Similarly highly complex questions of maintaining acceptable social and behavioural standards within an environment pose dilemmas which must be responded to by approaches predicated upon positive choice and decision-making. It only takes an apparently benign situation to occur, that of doing nothing by default, for worst practice to begin to develop, and from there institutionalised decay and the associated neglect of individuals will inevitably follow. There are too many examples of this pattern for it not to be the case. It is precisely for this reason that it becomes imperative to manage care situations actively.

Whilst our students' lists are by no means exhaustive, and include qualitatively different issues, they are representative of the functions which we have seen in the literature. We can compare them with examples taken from inspections, enquiries and research studies into living environments, and perhaps acknowledge that they are a product of both the formal and informal systems within institutions. All examples of sustained good practice derive from highly developed philosophical and practice backgrounds. They do not happen by chance. However, unless systems are specifically adopted to avoid it, institutions with basically best practice models will always develop some aspects of worst practice. In contrast, whilst the worst institutions have the potential to exhibit some positive or acceptable facets of practice (though this cannot serve to protect them from criticism), all it takes for worst practice to prevail is to do nothing.

It is not difficult to think of reasons for explaining how worst practice can arise (from 'I was only doing what I was told', to laying the blame at the feet of 'management' or resourcing inadequacies). Enquiry after enquiry has drawn attention to the fact that staff have not challenged within institutions behaviour which, if witnessed by the very same people in an outside context, would frequently be viewed as unacceptable. Equally, in the inevitable stresses of living with other people's tempestuous and chaotic lives (as well as coping with our own . . .), we can all, from time to time, react irrationally and in ways which we later might regret. The persons who would willingly accommodate exposure of their vulnerabilities as a common facet of their working lives, subjecting their selves to scrutiny and analysis, is rare indeed. Yet this can be a normative occurrence when working within an institutional setting. We have to, therefore, temper our judgement with pragmatism, but in all instances ensure that our practice is mature and underpinned by an unimpeachable values base. Perhaps the most fundamental lesson which can be learned from this type of scrutiny of the literature is the importance of learning to share power, and ensuring that embedded systems which are capable of overriding personal predilections are firmly in place. In Chapter 4 we explore one way of initiating this process by considering the matter of management perspectives within the health and social care institutions.

# Models of managing, quality and regulation

**4**

The wider context

Stakeholder/user perspectives

Development of models of quality

Conclusions

There can sometimes be a temptation, from the practitioner's point of view, to think of management as either someone else's problem or a matter of less importance than getting on with the job in hand. It is not difficult to think of circumstances in which the trials of our working worlds have been heaped upon 'management', sometimes objectified as 'the management'. In her introductory text, *Management in Social Work*, Coulshed (1990) wrote telling, initial chapters which should be read by all those who might be inclined to believe that management is not their business. One of her central themes is that 'our circles of activity ripple away from managing "me" at the core to managing others and then on to managing systems' (Coulshed, 1990, p. 1), and it is now generally acknowledged that the term 'management' must be applied to all types of work, since all posts include some degree of management function. This may be to do with operational management, sometimes to do with organisational management, and at all times it is mostly defined by hierarchy and organisational structure. From the management of one's own workload to human resources management, management matters touch all employees.

Whilst issues of personal strategies for personal management are a crucial part of working life (for example managing stress, learning to be assertive, time management), it is not our purpose to explore those issues here. However, although this chapter is not intended to become a substantive trawl of the management literature, it is helpful to begin with some background exploration of the forms of thinking which have led to the range of current influential perspectives. Therefore, we shall be looking at selected aspects of management theory with a view to providing a platform to explore developments in those aspects of the management function which have to do with issues of quality and regulation in the context of institutional living. Here again, the historical overview is important, since it enables us to trace the origins, and conceptual basis, of current day developments. Within this review we include approaches to quality assurance as one expression of effective organisational operation.

## The wider context

Management theory developed within a wider industrial, economic and political context, and there are classically three major strands to the development of modern management theories. The first approach is known as the 'scientific' school of management thinking, which includes the work of the sociologist Weber (1985), and Fayol (1841–1925, published 1988), a French mining engineer who defined management for the first time. This was concerned with conceptualising hierarchical orders and frameworks, within which were located positions of authority, and developing rational descriptions of how functions were carried out. In this approach the structures and tasks of bureaucracy were more important than the specific individuals, who both comprised the former and performed the latter. This theoretical approach is frequently termed the 'prescriptive' approach, since it is essentially interested in prescribing models for implementation rather than understanding how people really operate within organisations. This is not to imply that the writers associated with this group were not conscious of the role of people within organisations, but rather that they were more interested in the technical and mechanical aspects of how organisations functioned.

The second approach is usually referred to as the 'human relations' school of management. Here writers such as Maslow (1970), McGregor (1985) and Likert (1987) were much more concerned with exploring the notion that people, rather than structures, make organisations what they are. Maslow's well-known work on the hierarchy of human need was related to organisational function and satisfying needs within the work setting. McGregor developed his 'XY' theory, which explored the opposing assumptions about imposed motivation versus self-motivation in the work force. He classified workers as those who either innately disliked work and had to be controlled and directed (theory X), or saw work as a natural activity and were self-directed and committed to their work (theory Y). Likert developed a series of management systems which accommodated the view that both organisations and workers operated across a spectrum which ranged from the rigid to the participative. There were also other writers such as Follet (see Coulshed, 1990), who recognised that organisations functioned dynamically, with both horizontal and vertical strands of formal and informal relationships, and who acknowledged the significance of effective communications systems.

The third of the classical approaches is to be found in the work of writers who have applied systemic thinking to management and organisational theory. Originally developed from the physical sciences, this approach takes the notions of macro systems, systems and subsystems and their relationships one to another. It acknowledges that systems can be organic or mechanical and that the boundaries around them, whether they be open, closed or permeable, will have effects and consequences. Organisational structures and relationships can be analysed and developed through systemic methodology (Burns and Stalker, 1961; Lawton and Rose, 1994).

All of this, then, forms a substantial part of the background to how we view management today. However, there is also a fourth strand which includes writers such as Peters and Waterman (1982), Peters (1987) and Handy (1989) and which acknowledges more centrally the confusions and problems which must be addressed in order to enable organisations to work more effectively. It is worth our while devoting a little more time to the work of this group of writers, since it will form a useful basis for our consideration of issues of quality and regulation.

## CHAOS VERSUS REGULATION

It is scarcely surprising, in the light of the above material, to find managers with fixed management approaches who align themselves to specific theories. And it is probably tautological to suggest that most managers will adopt a model of management which fits, rather than contradicts, their own characteristic styles. However, it was within this context that Peters and Waterman's (1982) classic work *In Search of Excellence* was presented as a distillation of lessons from some of America's best known companies. It offered a rational model, not of the Weberian variety but one which took the stance that if a problem was identified, then resources should be put into it to get things fixed. The book is heavily orientated to all things American, and to a non-American reader can appear somewhat alien in its language, examples and general presentation. However, distilled to the essence of its messages, a valid and contemporary perspective continues to emerge.

The authors identify eight basic characteristics of excellent management practice. These are the capacity for:

- **Dealing with ambiguity and paradox:** these have to be managed. Old theories (management orthodoxies) were attractive because they were straightforward and *not* laden with ambiguity or paradox. The essence of managing complexity is to acknowledge that there are rarely simple, single solutions.
- **Sustaining a bias for action:** the organisation has to be action-oriented. There must be organisational flexibility, the capacity to experiment, to simplify rather than complicate (it was in this sense that they promoted the notion of the 'one page' memo).
- **Keeping a closeness to the customer:** there should be an obsession with service and quality, organisations should listen to their service-users. Implicit to this notion is the idea that we must be responsive to customers (however they might be defined, an issue to which we shall return when we consider the meaning of the term 'stakeholder').
- **Promoting autonomy and entrepreneurship:** creativity should be valued, and failure tolerated. This does not mean that 'anything goes', but that organisations should encourage a cultural embedding of creativity, and all which that implies, that is properly supported within supervisory structures. In other words, that it is ultimately the organisation, rather than the individual, which assumes responsibility for any risks taken.
- **Achieving productivity through people:** a common language should be

fostered, there should be less structuring/layering, and incoming managing should be socialised into best practice. There should be no undue reliance on structures and systems, the bedrock of 'scientific management', but a recognition that it is the way in which people operate which determines the effective functioning of the organisation.

- **Be hands on, values driven:** explicit attention must be paid to values, at all levels and at all times. Coulshed coined the phrase 'virtuous management', by which she meant that people should not desert their professional values when moving into a management arena: the term 'principled management' is also used to mean the same thing.
- **'Sticking to the knitting':** doing what you are there for and questioning diversification. This is an intriguing choice of words, but the message is instantly clear: keeping your prime function uppermost. The maintenance of simple, lean structures can facilitate this approach.
- **Maintaining simultaneous loose/tight properties:** maintaining the capacity to be fluid or disciplined where appropriate enables organisations to be 'market sensitive', or responsive. In this way, services are able to adapt to changing circumstances: there are no organisations which do not change, and it is far better to manage change proactively and creatively rather than reactively.

This range of ideas posed a fundamental challenge to the orthodox management approaches. The combination of creative thinking and idiosyncratic language assured the book a reputation as a completely radical text. It can be a salutary exercise to apply the eight principles to organisations with which we are familiar. No theory can ever be a perfect fit and it is often argued, particularly within the health and welfare professions, that the commercial organisations from which the book sprang cannot properly be used as a basis for comparison with other types of organisations. However, it is a specious position to imagine that health and social care are somehow entirely removed from the world of industry and commerce. The mechanisms of welfare pluralism which were introduced by the Thatcher governments have ensured that the marketplace characteristics of that world are equally embedded in public service organisations; and in any event independent sector organisations are by definition operating within the market processes of the commercial world. Notions of the 'new managerialism' are in danger of becoming polarised by the extremes of perspectives. There is one position which sees the introduction of a managerialist approach as little more than a return to 'Victorian' autocratic processes, whilst another sees it as an essential component in upgrading the efficiency of service delivery processes. This polarisation can equally be seen as a clash between ideologies and practices, where the person concerned with the delivery of services is accused of not being sufficiently aware of resource and other structural constraints, whilst the manager of services is seen as not understanding the operational implications of face-to-face work with service-users. This is an inevitably artificial divide, but one where the overlap of role boundary is central. The introduction of the role of care management in community care can be seen as an attempt to bridge this divide, as might some models of keyworking, though whilst some practitioners might see this as a welcome empowering development (Irvine and Gertig, 1998) others have seen it as a means of limiting and deprofessionalising their work (Thompson in Adams, Dominelli and Payne, 1998).

It is not difficult to identify concrete examples from the world of institutional living which match the descriptors of Peters and Waterman's eight characteristics. Even the overt language of the business environment, for example 'entrepreneurship' and 'values driven', does not appear too out of place. Indeed, the inventories of best and worst practice reviewed in our previous chapter provide clear illustrations of the issues which need to be managed well, and which embrace everything from 'ambiguity and paradox' to the maintenance of 'simultaneous loose/tight fit properties'. Issues such as care versus control, and dependency versus independency come to mind. Neither is it difficult to identify specific examples which might be common across a range of particular practice settings. For example, what approaches are taken to the management of wandering/absconding; or behaviour requirements, whether they be non-compliance with a treatment regime or the internal rules of safe conduct?

In a later work, entitled *Thriving on Chaos* (1987), Peters developed some of the earlier themes. He argued that there was no such thing as a successful company and that nothing was safe. At first reading this seems to be an uncharacteristically nihilistic statement from Peters. What he meant was that nothing was ever solid or substantial for all time and he suggested prescriptions for a world turned upside down, as he saw it, in the rapidly changing political and economic environment of the 1980s. It may have been a coincidence that the book was published on the same day in October 1987 as the Wall Street stock market crash, but this book was in many ways a product of its times. Peters' prescriptions were that it was essential to acknowledge the need to revolutionise management through being proactive in:

• an obsession with responsiveness to customers;
• constant innovation;
• working in partnership;
• leadership that loves (rather than fights) change;
• maintaining control by simple support systems.

These themes will appear as familiar echoes from the Peters and Waterman text. However, they are argued in the context of a necessity to pursue fast-paced innovation and to attain and maintain 'undreamed of' flexibility by empowering people. Once again it might appear as a surprise to those who are unfamiliar with this literature. Here we have examples drawn from the world of business management which are person-centred. The fact that it might appear surprising is an indicator of just how separated the two areas once were, and demonstrates the extent to which the two different worlds of work share much in common. The bullet points identified above could be embraced in their entirety by the health and social care professions. Indeed, as we discuss later on, the regulatory mechanisms applied to social and nursing care are increasingly adopting such approaches.

Another influential writer who developed the theme of the 'world turned upside down' was Handy. In *The Age of Unreason* (1989) he explored perspectives of individual and organisational activity through the three headings of changing, working and living. His target audience was those who worked in, and managed, organisations: and a major theme was that, far from the future being inevitable, we could influence it if we wanted to do so. Interestingly, Handy identified differential cultural characteristics of change. He felt that Europeans looked back to the best of their experiences and changed as little of it as possible, whilst Americans looked forward and wanted to change as much as they could.

Handy's basic themes were that:

- current changes are always different from past changes;
- the little changes make the biggest difference;
- discontinuous change (i.e. change which does not follow on naturally from what preceded it) requires discontinuous thinking, even if it seems absurd at first sight.

He also proposed that major change in organisations seemed to follow a predictable sequence of:

- fright: the possibility of take-over or collapse;
- new faces: new people brought in at the top;
- new questions: investigating old ways and new options;
- new structures: the break-up of old patterns and clubs, new talent given scope;
- new goals and standards: the new organisation sets itself new aims and targets.

Once again, it can be instructive to test these ideas out on our own experiences of organisations. Handy was a thinker who recognised the impact that changes in demography and working practices were having on both organisations and their workforces. He noted the trends in a move away from labour intensive manufacturing and towards service industries and knowledge-based organisations. Indeed, it can be said that in developing his theory of learning he was pre-empting by 10 years the lifelong learning approach of education for work of the late 1990s. More specifically, from a management theory point of view, he developed a model of the new organisations which were needed to keep pace with the changing world. Handy proposed the 'shamrock' organisation; characterised by a smaller core with a contractual fringe, a flexible labour force and the customer undertaking more of the product-related responsibilities. He also wrote of the federal organisation, a variety of groups allied together because of common issues. These themes are very much resonant with developments in the provision of both health and social care. Examples are: the increased use of employment agency staffing and temporary/part-time contracts, the reduced scale of established permanent workforces, and an increasing responsiveness to consumer/user demand.

In *The Empty Raincoat* (1994) Handy returned to these issues in an attempt to develop a meta-theoretical, quasi-pragmatic philosophical approach to his recognition that much of his earlier observation had become a reality. He had moved on from writing essentially about the world of work to writing about how to reconcile a successful working life with a successful personal life. In many ways this was an example of the management literature turning full circle. For those of us concerned with living and working in institutions, these two aspects of life are both separate and inseparable in equal turns. However, one of the most significant ideas which we can extract from this school of thinking is the discipline of discontinuous thinking: learning to turn our known world upside down and thinking the previously unthinkable. In *The Empty Raincoat*, itself a metaphor for the need to be more than an external shell, Handy ends by relating the story of a remarkably effective piece of creative thinking. It is the tale of how one of his relatives introduced the system of pre-paid, flat-rate postage to anywhere in the country, where previously all post had been charged cash-on-delivery according to distance travelled and weight. This guiding principle of our postal services does not seem at all remarkable to us today, but in the nineteenth century it was revolutionary.

It is possible to identify equally revolutionary past innovations into institutional beliefs (we have already identified the Victorian principle of less-eligibility), but more difficult to project them from the present into the future. Illich's (1971) call for institutional revolution was in considerable measure his response to a recognition that in his view the great meta-institutions of the twentieth century were failing society. If we were to examine our own areas of institutional operation – for instance from nursing homes for older people, residential homes for children and young people, hospices, bail hostels, psychiatric wards – finding practical and effective solutions to the criticisms which we might raise is far more problematic than identifying the criticisms in the first instance. It is here that, arguably, this literature fails us. It takes us so far on the journey, but so often runs out of usable ideas to employ in our search for improvement. The fact of calling for a need to be creative is qualitatively very different from the activity of creativity itself. Nevertheless, practitioners such as those identified as positive exemplars of institutional practice in Chapter 3 were largely successful by virtue of their challenging of the prevailing orthodoxes, as well as their bringing of considerable creativity to bear on their work.

In their preoccupation with developing a responsive organisation whose sole justification for existence is to put the customer first, writers such as Peters and Handy have embodied the essential principles which underpin approaches to quality and regulation in institutional living. There *are* ideas that can seem revolutionary today, and one of the ways in which we can apply lessons from this literature is to open our minds to new or challenging possibilities. There can be a curious disjuncture between knowing something in our heads, and putting it into operation. For example, part of our shared values system is to value human dignity, self-worth and self-determination; yet there are times when we do not stop to think about how actions can impact on the rights of others for whose care we are responsible. In writing this book it is part of our aspiration to encourage the reader positively to apply these values, rather than simply to know them.

## Stakeholder/user perspectives

Before moving on to examine the more specific literature which links management and quality systems, it is important to say a little about the role and conceptualisation of the 'customer'. As we have already suggested, there is no great difficulty in associating the activities of social and health care organisations with those of organisations with different end services or products. Not only has the general principle been accepted within welfare organisations, but there are also now familiar examples of where the specific language has been imported, for example the use of 'customer service' designations for sections of social services departments which deal with standards and complaints issues. If the persuasive weight of accepted 'virtuous' management theory now is that people, rather than systems, are more important to successful functioning, then we can both learn from others' experiences and teach others from our own. The paradox is that a quality product has both commonalities and dissimilarities with a quality service. We shall see in the next section that quality is not intangible, can be measured or assessed, and its pursuit must become a central activity. However, in the first instance there is considerable debate about how to define the 'customer'. At its simplest, the customer is the person who is the end-user, the one who 'buys' the product. In the institutional group living application it could be argued that this is obviously the resident or patient, using whatever local terminology as is appropriate. However, it does not take much analysis to begin to develop a sense that this might be both simplistic and inadequate. Of course the resident is, in this sense, the customer; but equally there may be a range of other customers, for instance a carer, or a relative who may not be a hands-on carer, but might have other responsibilities (for example an absent parent or the holder of enduring powers of attorney).

Very easily we see that the word 'customer' is not necessarily always helpful. The term 'stakeholder' has been adopted in a variety of contexts in recognition of the fact that a potentially wide range of people will have an interest in a particular service. And it is not without significance to notice just how often the term is used in the literature without any attempt to define its parameters, quite often being used as a synonym for customer or service-user. If the customer is always right, and needs to be listened and responded to, we are immediately beset by potentially conflicting and competing demands. A problem with moving into the stakeholder lexicon is that it might acknowledge multiple interest, but also renders it difficult to meet their varying demands. Nevertheless, it is important that the complexities of the relationships are acknowledged and efforts made to satisfy them.

Wilmot (1997), writing about the ethics of community care, makes a helpful contribution to this dilemma by distinguishing between constituency,

consumers and stakeholders. Within this ethics context, he defines constituency as the grouping (in our case, perhaps the welfare profession/
industry) which the organisation represents and which gives it legitimacy;
consumers as those for whom the services are provided (perhaps the resident,
or other service-user); and stakeholders as the various other organisations and
individuals affected by, or involved with, the organisation. (This is more
problematic for us: does it include carers and families, or is it specifically other
involved professionals, etc.?) However even this model offers only a degree of
clarification since at best, as our examples demonstrate, there is no universally
acknowledged definition and at worst it can lead to the development of a
multilayered level of complexity. Perhaps what is most helpful about
Wilmot's selection of language is that it can serve to reinforce to us the
importance of maintaining the profile of the consumer as principal
'customer'. By the same token, however, the views of those with other
legitimate interests in the organisation cannot be ignored.

## Development of models of quality

Whilst forms of statutory regulation have long existed, the arenas of welfare
and health provision were relative latecomers in adopting modern concepts of
quality regulation in respect of service provision. The public service ethos of
health and welfare in the 1970s and 1980s eventually learned from models
previously developed in industry and commerce. It is arguable that the
pressures to regulate the increasingly commercialised, contract-driven nature
of these services has been a key driver in this respect.

Modern constructions of quality regulation instruments began with the
development of large-scale manufacturing processes in the post-Second
World War era. As part of the drive both to become more efficient and to
deliver in accordance with customer requirements, manufacturing organisations needed to develop mechanisms which would be more effective in
ensuring quality outputs. In the first instance, systems of quality control were
developed. These systems essentially involved the inspection of products at
points in the manufacturing process. However, it became apparent that this
was a wasteful approach, since by the time any flaws were identified,
considerable resources had already been employed to produce what had
become a redundant product. It could be argued that 'rota' visits of elected
members to local authority residential homes fall within this approach; so
might the presentation of meals which are not eaten because residents do not
like them. Irrespective of however sophisticated the systems might have
become, the capacity of this form of 'policing' to make any significant impact
on the general levels of functioning was extremely limited, and issues
identified through such a process were liable to become externally located
rather than internally owned.

In response to developing market conditions in the 1980s, and particularly
as a result of the success of Japanese manufacturing companies in European
markets, quality assurance procedures were developed. This approach

redefined quality as being everyone's responsibility, rather than that of a handful of specifically dedicated staff who themselves had no part in the production process. In this approach emphasis moves away from the output and towards the effectiveness of the systems of production. If all the systems can be assured to work, then the finished output must inevitably be quality assured to the required standards of production. Tools which were developed as part of this approach include quality circles, where small groups of workers meet locally with a view to enhancing the quality of their immediate work through an exchange of ideas. Quality assurance systems have, in turn, led to the development of an approach known as Total Quality Management or TQM, which delivers a systematic way of ensuring that organised activities happen in the way that they are planned. These developments in quality assurance are well documented both in terms of industry and the caring professions (Crosby, 1979; Donabedian, 1980; Ellis, 1988; Lock, 1990), and have led to the introduction within the United Kingdom of firstly British and then international quality standards. These standards have been applied to welfare services, especially institutional service. There also exist a number of bespoke packages (for examples see Kerruish and Smith, 1993; Kellaher, 1992; Allen, 1995).

## REGULATION, QUALITY, AND INSTITUTIONAL CARE

A Joseph Rowntree Foundation study (Day, Klein and Redmayne, 1996) explored the question 'why regulate' in respect of residential care for older people, but the overall findings are transferable across user groups. It makes the important point that many of the business-based reasons for regulation do not apply. For example, there is no need to control private monopolies *pro bono publico* though it might be added now that, with the growth of private sector companies operating in that sector, this may well become an issue. There is also the contrary view that the public sector is a monopoly and operates within a privileged context controlling, as it does, the mechanisms of regulation. Similarly, the report argues that 'models of behaviour which may fit customers in the marketplace . . . may be inappropriate when applied to residential care' (p. 7). Overall, a persuasive case is made for regulation; not, however, without differentiating between regulating (and inspecting) for risk reduction on the one hand and ensuring the quality of the provision on the other. Day and colleagues suggest that there are a number of regulatory models: policing versus consultancy (i.e. enforcement versus partnership); rules versus discretion; and stringency versus accommodation (characterised by a pedantic, trivialising approach to regulation rather than understanding the complexity of some of the problems). Whilst a balance undoubtedly needs to be struck across these approaches, there are a great many difficulties, for example between avoiding an adversarial approach but ensuring that collusion does not occur.

The idea of regulation leads us into thinking about quality issues and Allen (1995) suggests that there are three phrases which offer a framework for understanding the idea of quality: 'quality assurance cycle', 'standard setting',

and 'audit instruments'. We shall be looking more specifically at the latter in the final chapter of this book, and for the present shall build upon the ground already explored in relation to the management of quality. Although we have argued that quality assurance is a concept which is transferable from industry to welfare, this does not mean to say that it is always easily done. The approach offers more formalised systems for 'opening-up' care, but also presents its own assumptions which need to be challenged. Whilst there are undoubtedly complex production issues in the manufacturing industry, the unpredictability of personal characteristics in the welfare 'industry' is the very essence of its day-to-day activity. The introduction of *Home Life* (Care Centre for Policy on Ageing, 1984), *A Better Home Life* (Care Centre for Policy on Ageing, 1996) and the Wagner Report (1988) heralded the setting of wide-ranging identifiable standards within the context of a quality assurance style of approach. In due course the statutory requirements of the Children Act 1989 and the NHS and Community Care Act of 1990 ensured that local authority social services departments set up inspection units which were to regulate standards and investigate complaints.

However, although the underlying philosophy of the Department of Health acknowledged the centrality of quality assurance (*Inspecting for Quality* [1991]; *The Inspection of the Complaints Procedures in LASSD* [1993]), the major function of regulation had more in common with a quality control approach than one of quality assurance. Similarly the substantial number of standards guidance documents issued by the Department of Health during the same period and later, and which covered a wide range of service-user groups, were very much concerned with articulating the required standards to be imposed. There was little on offer which addressed systems for the implementation and maintenance of appropriate standards within the care settings. Indeed, there remains at the present time no effective, widely available model aimed at establishing quality assurance principles. There is, of course, a huge literature on good practice and institutional living which we have already, in part, reviewed. But the mechanisms of quality assurance as developed and embraced by industry do not have their counterparts which permeate welfare provision. It is for this very reason that we began our journey into writing this book. However, it is becoming apparent that certain sectors, for example the independent sector which provides residential and nursing care for older people, are increasingly introducing quality assurance mechanisms on a voluntary basis and more may in due course (partly as a result of EU regulatory initiatives) be required to do so.

Even though there may not be extensively established models of practice, there is the beginning of a ground swell, in part precipitated by the Wagner Report, to develop quality within the care environment in a more proactive sense. The Caring in Homes Initiative was commissioned by the Department of Health as a follow-up to Wagner and has been reported on in detail by Youll and McCourt-Perring (1993). This initiative created research and development programmes which included an internal review system for residential homes and the development of links between the local community and residential care homes. The adoption by many private sector homes of International

Standards Organization (ISO) standards indicates the search for usable tools. A study by Raynes *et al.* (1994) which looked at cost in relation to quality of care does, however, caution that the use of process measures of quality does not necessarily mean that they have a beneficial impact on the wellbeing of service-users.

Peace *et al.* (1997) make reference to the movement from quality control to quality assurance in the monitoring of residential and nursing care home environments, and also refer to the changing emphasis as a move from bureaucratic to person-centred models of regulation. What they acknowledge is a range of instruments which take account of the people involved, and in particular the resident. They cite the Rowntree Foundation study by O'Kell in 1995 which identified eleven quality assurance systems in operation, drawing attention to the fact that most of them did not develop a substantial focus on the relationships between quality of care and quality of life as experienced by the people involved, especially the residents. Two quite different approaches can be seen in the systems developed by Kerruish and Smith (1992), *Developing Quality Residential Care: A User Led Approach* and Allen (1995), *Surviving the Registration and Inspection Process: A Guide for Care Home Owners and Managers*. Both of these publications take the form of loose-leaf manuals. It is not our purpose here to undertake a detailed critique of them, but rather to present them as different exemplars of this type of material.

Kerruish and Smith's model was based on a King's Fund initiative and is broadly aimed at operational managers in health and social care residential services. The basis for the system is derived from a previous project which was aimed at discovering residents' perspectives and developing a user led approach to creating quality assurance tools. The substantive sections of the manual cover the quality framework (relationships, equality and empowerment, choice and control, developing skills, community integration) monitoring methods, training and guidelines for implementing each method, processes for developing a quality framework, and the relevance of the framework to service commissioners. Thus the subtitle 'user led' relates partly to the origins of the material, and partly to a process which is designed to procure responses from service-users. The various methods of implementation include exercises for training and awareness development, guidance and facilitation notes, and handouts to stimulate discussion or for use as further reading. Methods for obtaining responses include creating a service-user group, questionnaires, review of specific services and facilities, and reference to a residents association. This is a complex and sophisticated instrument which also offers details about other relevant packages and how to access them. The significance of its approach is that the material is research based, albeit on a single user group (people with long-term mental health problems who had been discharged from hospital to residential or nursing care), and has a user-derived focus.

In contrast, Judy Allen's guide is aimed primarily at assisting the owner or manager in understanding the registration process, how to manage inspections, the methods and reasons for record keeping, the importance of networking, how to plan education and training for staff, and how to

introduce quality measures. This then is a procedural 'bible' for home managers which in passing locates procedures in notions of good practice. And Allen is anxious to point out that its purpose is to facilitate and improve, not to offer the manager tips on how to avoid their regulatory responsibilities. Interestingly, she refers to Kerruish and Smith's manual as an audit document, which is in essence only a partial description. However, it is significant that Allen sees staff training and the introduction of quality assurance mechanisms as going 'beyond the basics'. It is a debatable point, even within the declared aims of the manual, as to whether satisfying the registration and inspection requirements is a necessary preliminary to establishing quality care, or whether the provision of quality care ensures the meeting of the requirements. No doubt the ultimate reality is a cyclical one. However, it is a reflection on the registration and inspection approach to delivering services that embedded quality systems are more likely to be seen as a second order activity.

Another dimension which these two examples highlight is the contrast between externally and internally managed systems. A criticism which can be levelled at externally monitored systems is that they provide perhaps little more than a temporal 'snapshot' at the time of monitoring (however important that snapshot might be) and do not necessarily therefore exert anything other than a surface influence upon the care environment. They might not even be seen by operational day-to-day practitioners as part of everyday practice. For example, it might be that systems are unimpeachably in place: procedures manuals duly written and filed, or recording systems maintained in good order. However, as a sole approach, this tendency to focus on the physical and environmental levels of provision may militate against addressing the quality of the lived experience. The two are not inevitably mutually exclusive, but externally imposed systems may create a limited sense of vision. The controls are very important for the policing of minimum standards, but it is unfortunate if the baseline measurements and their associated systems are set solely to prevent standards of practice falling below the unacceptable. What is required alongside the minimum standards safeguard is the adoption of a process which will also encourage and enable the best possible of standards to develop and flourish. Whilst it can undoubtedly be a demanding task to ensure that mechanical processes such as control of medicines and food hygiene are systematised, it is a challenge of an altogether different level to ensure that the higher order needs of personal fulfilment are met.

## Conclusions

The White Paper, *Modernising Social Services* (Department of Health, 1998) contains a substantive section on regulation (Chapter 4), with proposals to increase both the range of service provision to be regulated and the extent of that regulation. In determining the level of regulation to which any provision might be exposed, it suggests that providers will:

be assessed in relation to various factors, including past history, previous concerns or complaints ... Other quality assurance mechanisms – such as independent accreditation schemes – could also be taken into account in determining the level of attention paid to the particular provider.                                    (Cmnd 4169, para 4.54)

However, we would argue, as do Peace *et al.* (1997), that the adoption of a self-regulation approach should become an imperative. This theme was taken up by Burgner (1996) who acknowledged the contribution of the statutory inspection units in regulating social services, but also recognised that the quality of service cannot be easily regulated from the outside, and that it is much more likely to be achieved if it is genuinely owned by providers. However, we should like to nudge a little further in that direction and suggest that it should equally, in Wilmot's (1997) parlance, be owned by constituency, consumer and stakeholder alike. We are not convinced that the case for first-level, externally imposed inspection is persuasive in ensuring standards. There is substantial evidence emerging to indicate that self-regulation can produce a change of attitude at service-delivery levels, leading to a greater acceptance of responsibility for setting and maintaining standards. It is much more useful to the effective management of institutions for staff to experience standards maintenance as part and parcel of their everyday activity, rather than as an episodic event which interrupts the norm. Equally, what is true for the service providers is true for all parties involved. It will, of course, always be necessary for enforcement procedures to be in place but they should not, as is the case at present, be the first and sometimes only line of approach.

Finally, as we hope has become clear by now, we are interested in the impact which such mechanisms have on the daily practice of staff and the lived experience of the service-users. We believe that there is a gap between most imposed systems and the reality of care. If self-regulation is to become meaningful it needs to reflect a process which ensures ongoing good practice, and it therefore becomes self-evident that either good practice must coexist with self-regulatory instruments, or the instrument itself must be developed to become a tool for implementing good practice. This is no arcane utterance or semantically circular argument, for we have already considered the possibility that all that is required for bad practice to prevail is to do nothing. Therefore, it becomes imperative to ensure that there are processes in place which will introduce and reinforce good practice.

# Models of working – professional practice

Practice does not happen in a theoretical vacuum – it happens in the context of a range of different models held explicitly and implicitly by practitioners, service-users and those who do not experience care delivery, but who comment on it in a range of capacities. Models may be multiple and may conflict with each other; they may have an internal coherence which does not bear up to external scrutiny, or they may be so vague and covert that they are only glimpsed occasionally. It is not the intention of this chapter to divert into an examination of the minutiae of specific models, but to identify that a range does exist and to encourage the readers to contextualise their own practice within a conceptually-based model or matrix of models. In many respects we shall be dealing with abstract models and therefore, in the first instance, shall focus on what we mean by 'models'.

## What is a model?

It is probably worth revisiting some definitions and ideas about what a model is, and what sort of use it may have in professional practice, otherwise the discussion feels very abstract and irrelevant. Sometimes, models of practice are presented in esoteric ways, which makes them difficult to connect up to everyday working, and sometimes models are so vague and woolly that it is difficult to think about them critically – they can feel like meaningless slogans. At a very basic level, a model is a way of thinking about or representing something in reality. An example often given is that of the London Underground map – it is a model of the system which shows you how to get around it, but does not correspond to it in any geographical sense – the distances between stations in real life are not equivalent to the distances on the diagram. The problem with the Underground map as an example, however, is that a railway system does not equate with ideas about care – a tangible concrete thing such as the Tube is, we feel, quite different to the processes of care. In making this distinction, however, we are already doing some modelling – describing care as a process and not a concrete object, but we might want to hold on to the idea of care as a system where, like the Underground, different components are linked up.

We need to move on a bit from leaving the model as 'care is a process'. This doesn't help us to discuss what the process is for, what sort of process it is, what is involved, or what happens at the end (if there is one). This is where the utility of developing models becomes more apparent. If we can be a bit clearer about what we think care is, then we can start to examine it and critique it. We can start to see where the anomalies lie, where the logic takes us, what is not accounted for in the model, and so on. Earlier in this book we sketched out some models of institutions, although we did not call them this. There were ideas about the institution as a sanctuary, as a place of punishment, and as a warehouse, to name but a few of the models that have been adopted over the years. Those who worked and lived in institutions, and those who campaigned for change, used these models as ways of understanding what was going on, why it was going on, and what the outcomes were. Understanding a model doesn't necessarily mean supporting it, and there is the possibility that different models are noticed or supported by different people at different times – it is likely, for example, that those who worked in institutions and those who lived in them had very different ideas about them. They may have accepted the prevailing ideas about the function of institutions, but they may have disagreed about the ethics of these goals or the way in which they were carried out. Working out where these disagreements might lie is helped by being clear about the models that people are using.

Perhaps a word of caution is needed here about trying to be too precise about a model. Attempts in some professions, nursing being one notable example, to develop models in a very precise form have, by and large, been unhelpful to practice because of the length and complexity of these attempts. Moving from broad principles of nursing, through concepts of health to values in relationships with patients, nursing models have gone on to elaborate these ideas, drawing on a vast (and sometimes incompatible) range of research and theory to flesh out this structure, often to disastrous effect. Trying to develop a universal model which is applicable to every context and client usually involves a degree of complexity which renders the model unwieldy and cumbersome. In view of this, we are not attempting to provide elaborate descriptions of models (indeed some of them have not been precisely thought through or articulated), but simply to provide an outline of their basic principles, what they portray practice as being about, how they describe it as happening and what sort of qualities or skills are necessary for it.

We also argue that all models of practice are caught up with ideas about what institutions are for, and how people feel that societies should deal with people in institutions. Models are, at least partly, expressions of the aspirations of a society – they are about how it sees itself. Societies which see themselves as liberal and caring have different ideas about institutions and how they should operate, than societies who aspire to an ethos which is about being orderly and efficient, for example. Some of the ideas about institutions which were voiced in Victorian times, for example, seem to fit with ideas that society had about itself as a virtuous and industrious community, which was rigorous in its adherence to discipline and regulation. In this sense, the practitioner acts as a proxy for the rest of society – they do on behalf of society what those people feel that they would do themselves, or would like to think that they do themselves.

This puts the practitioner in an interesting position, as a go-between for the service-user and the wider society. Acting as a proxy for the general wishes or vague ideas of society is fraught with problems, as many practitioners have found when what seemed like reasonable actions according to their training or organisational framework have been vilified in the press. This type of tension makes the clarification of models of practice even more important – it opens up these ideas to scrutiny and debate within the profession, the organisation and in the culture in which they operate.

## Practice as benevolent charity

This model of practice has a long history and remains powerful today – we see it in media stories about 'angels of mercy' and selfless workers for the underprivileged. The institution is seen as a haven or sanctuary in which the disadvantaged can be given succour. The corresponding qualities of practice are that it should be entirely positive in its actions and seek only the good of the service-user.

There are, of course, many complexities left unexamined at this level of analysis. What, for example, do we mean by 'the good of the service-user'? The benevolence model tends to take this for granted and does not deal with cases where this good is in question. It covers adequately a dilemma of a straightforward nature, for example where a patient in a hospital needs water, but the nurse is about to go on a coffee break. The benevolence model would clearly expect the nurse to delay the coffee break in order to get the water.

Where the conflict is not simply between the good of the staff and the good of the service-users, but is about what we call good and how we could identify it, the picture becomes more complicated. If a service-user wants a particular service or facility which practitioners feel might not be appropriate, indeed may be detrimental, then where does the benevolence model take us? To take two examples, a child in a residential home may want to make unsupervised visits to a parent who has been abusive in the past, or a hospital patient may request high doses of painkillers that can have damaging side effects. In one formulation, good might be defined as whatever the service-user wants – the visit to the parent or increased dosage of drugs. In another, it might be defined as whatever the experts think is best – avoiding parental abuse or drug side effects. The first formulation can rest on a number of assumptions: that granting wishes is in itself a good thing because it respects rights to self-determination (for a fuller discussion of rights see Chapter 7), or that there is no expertise greater than that of the service-user – the child or the patient knows what he or she wants and needs better than anyone else. The second version privileges the expert opinion, and correspondingly devalues the view of the service-user: parental abuse or drug side effects are likely and would be very damaging. The differences between these two positions are vast, and the differences in the actions and outcomes that arise from them are correspondingly huge. We might, therefore, want to refine this model of practice to include two types of benevolence: client-centred and practitioner-centred.

To outline the differences between these two models in simplistic terms, the client-centred version would incorporate ideas of empowerment and rights, while the practitioner-centred model would be based on ideas of practitioner expertise and knowledge. In other words, client-centred benevolence, while not without its problems (as we discuss further on), carries some ideas of the primacy of the service-user, while practitioner-centred benevolence shifts the service-user slightly to one side, as someone who may be central in terms of a focus of activity, but marginalised in the business of deciding what form this activity should take. The differences between the two versions of the benevolence model are, therefore, vast, and this variation warns us not to take the model for granted.

The limitations of the benevolence model of practice are also evident when we think about how it portrays the practitioner and the qualities that he or she needs. Essentially, client-centred benevolence simply requires a kindly heart and a willingness to put the needs of others before those of the practitioner. It does not necessarily require knowledge; simply 'niceness'. How this quality should be identified or fostered in practitioners is not explored and, in many professions, where there is a concern to recruit 'the right sort' of person, these issues are left to intuition and luck – the idea is that you can tell who is 'caring' by some peculiar osmotic process, and similarly you can tell who isn't the right sort in the same way.

Practitioner-centred benevolence, because it is predicated on the expertise and knowledge of practitioners, has something more to say about the skills and knowledge needed by them; kindness is not enough. It does not, however, promote a particularly critical approach to knowledge, given that it has its foundations in ideas about the certainty of expertise – indeed too much doubt and debate would undermine the whole idea of the practitioner knowing best, and call into question the entire model of practice. If, in the examples given above, the practitioners wavered too much over the pros and cons of parental visits or increased doses then they would, in effect, be raising worrying concerns about the certainty of professional knowledge – that it does not provide clear-cut answers that can be trusted. The model of practitioner-centred benevolence, therefore, could be expected to promulgate a procedural form of knowledge – this is the right way to do things and the right decision to make. Forms of this type of knowledge crop up in a range of health and social care professions, for example clinical guidelines in medicine, and protocols and procedures in social care. These formulae for action promote the idea that there is one right way to do things, and are also easily connected to concerns about documenting and recording care accurately. If the procedure has been followed, as evidenced by records and notes, then the professionals are 'safe' in that they can be seen to have adhered to professional standards of practice. If anyone wishes to challenge the practice of the individual, then he or she must also take on the whole body of knowledge and practice norms that this individual has adopted. In the practitioner-centred benevolence model then, the notion of the goodwill of the practitioner is assumed (perhaps with a few lectures on ethics at the beginning of training), and this goodwill is seen as being expressed by adherence to accepted canons of practice knowledge.

The kindness of the practitioner, in both the client-centred and practitioner-centred models of benevolence, puts the service-users in a difficult position, especially if they want to rebel against whatever they are offered. Disagreeing with care, or refusing it, is much more difficult if it is offered under the auspices of benevolence, because then the rejection becomes personal – it is not simply a question of disagreeing with the strategies that the practitioner is suggesting, but also the motivation. To demur is to suggest that the practitioner does not have your best interests at heart. Additionally, the service-user becomes the beneficiary of benevolence with no opportunity to reciprocate. The vivid images that we have of recipients of charity, from frail older people to vulnerable children, do not include any notion that they might be giving something back to their benefactors – the traffic of kindness is entirely one way.

This denial of reciprocity does a number of things. It diminishes the service-user as an active agent and portrays him or her as entirely passive. This passivity is then taken as a rationale for privileging the expert's view, as this inability to act is taken as evidence of incompetence to act. A further idea is then brought into play, about the way in which the service-user should feel grateful to the practitioners for what they are providing, as he or she would not be able to cope without this assistance. Any rejection of care is then viewed not just as a difference in opinion, but as a moral failing – service-users are 'ungrateful', or 'awkward', or 'demanding'. If the child whose parental visit has been refused, or the patient whose painkillers have not been increased complains about the treatment, framing the actions of the professionals as benevolence allows the service-users' complaints to be framed as ignorance or rebellion, rather than simply a difference in opinion.

The conclusion of the client-centred and practitioner-centred benevolence models of practice, then, is that they put the service-user into a dependent position. In the practitioner-centred model this is perhaps more obvious, given the emphasis on expertise that it endorses and which, by definition, excludes the client or service-user. The client-centred notion of benevolence is perhaps more covert in the way that it promotes dependency through the emotional and moral imperatives that it embodies; for the service-user to be grateful for what is offered.

Interestingly, in view of the benign aspects of the model, it can also set up some tensions and conflicts between service-user and practitioner. In client-centred benevolence this can arise from the centrality of the client, which can 'demote' the practitioners to a position in which they are governed entirely by the client, and have little self-governance. Conversely, in practitioner-centred benevolence it is the client who is demoted. This demotion is not a necessary outcome for these models, but because the gloss of benevolence does not really address these possibilities, there are no cautions or safeguards visible. While benevolence may be workable where goals are shared, it does not deal with conflicts between parties. To return to the example of the nurse wanting a cup of coffee when a patient needs some water, we can see how in specific situations it would be appropriate to meet the patient's need first, and benevolence, particularly client-centred, would certainly push in this direction. For this to happen every day, or every time the nurse wants a coffee break, however, presents a different problem. Are we saying that client needs should always take precedence over staff needs and, if so, then how do staff sustain any degree of commitment or energy for their work when it clearly relegates their needs, even basic ones for rest, to the bottom of the heap?

This placing of staff and client needs in opposition to each other is a consequence of relying on simplistic notions of benevolence as a foundation or model of practice. Practitioner-centred benevolence does much the same, although in a slightly different way. With practitioner-centred benevolence, there are more routes out of the demoted position for staff. In the case of the coffee-needing nurse and the water-needing patient, a range of strategies can be used to justify the coffee break, couched in analyses of the patients' needs. Perhaps so much water is bad for them, perhaps they need to restrict their fluid intake, or perhaps the need can be re-interpreted as a manifestation of anxiety or attention seeking. In all of these arguments, the nurse has some plausible rationales, justifiable in terms of benevolence, which permit or even encourage the nurse to refuse a request for water (and thereby achieve a coffee break).

Another set of questions which can be asked about the benevolence models of practice is about their goals or endpoints. Having said that there is a global set of aspirations that care should be aimed at giving succour to the disadvantaged and needy, this leaves us with little to go on if we want to see if these goals have been achieved. The complexities involved in determining what is 'the good' and whose good it is are considerable. We have outlined possible conflicts between different views of what goals should be, and these are particularly apparent in practitioner-centred benevolence, where it can be anticipated that the practitioner's view might not coincide with that of the client. Even in client-centred benevolence, however, the problems of identifying goals are not avoided simply by referring to the service-users' preferences. There is a real question to be asked about the validity of these preferences, in terms of how they are arrived at. Client preferences may be determined by past experiences of limited services and restricted outcomes, in which case they may be over-modest and under-ambitious. They may be determined by images and anecdotes about ideal services, in which case they may be over-ambitious. They may be short term, and not cognisant of long-term implications, or based on limited information about the implications of their choices. The examples given above, of a child wanting to visit a parent, or a patient wanting more painkillers, could be interpreted as preferences which are based on limited information and understanding, although reflecting strong wishes and preferences.

These are real dilemmas, where the client choices may be too difficult to respond to because of limitations on services and resources, or may be too easy to respond to because they are minimal demands, or where the consequences of client choices may be harmful to themselves or others. Simply relying on a model of client-centred benevolence to direct responses is not enough, because the possibilities for the process to go wrong are significant. Relying on practitioner-centred benevolence, where the practitioner knows best, however, does not help in that it calls into question the validity of the practitioners' decisions – they may be just as problematic and, moreover, practitioner decisions tip the balance of power in ways with which we might not be comfortable.

These criticisms are useful ones to make about the notion of benevolence, which can often be accepted uncritically and, indeed, has been in the past. Notions of charity and duty, whereby those who were able to were exhorted to help those less fortunate than themselves, have not always been challenged, supported as they were by a whole range of religious and social arguments. Challenging these notions, however, does not mean that they should be entirely discarded. The idea of people helping each other seems a better option for society than the idea of everyone being only interested in their own welfare, and indeed some of the concerns that we express about society today are about such self-interest.

Perhaps the challenge, then, is to hold on to the idea of benevolence in the sense of people helping each other, but to model it in a way that is more critical and less complacent. As part of the process of doing this, it may also be useful to look at another option for a model of practice, one that presents a very different view of what practice is. Comparing these two models may lead us to a position which is more useful as a basis for practice that is reflective and supportive to service-users.

## Practice as control

Another model of practice in institutions is that of practice as being predominantly about containment and control. This has two forms: first, where control is expected of the institution, for example in prisons, and second, where control is assumed to happen but is disapproved of, for example in the literary depiction of a Victorian orphanage. This disapproval can range from an outright condemnation of control as being unjustified and simply wrong, to a timid regret for the necessity of control and some reservations about the way in which it is maintained.

The first version of practice as control, where it is expected of the institution, has in it some ideas about the service-user and the aim of practice which are worth examining. For someone to be deemed in need of control, it is usually the case that they have transgressed, or are thought to be likely to transgress some social rules or norms. These transgressions are not simply technical offences which interrupt the smooth running of society, but represent a threat to the foundations of this smooth running – a challenge to the principles and assumptions on which it is based. Similarly, controlling these transgressions is not simply a technical matter to be resolved purely through pragmatic and practical strategies, but is much more complex, involving some stance about values and carrying with it some form of moral force. There are then, some common sense or rational arguments about control, but also some more value-based arguments which contain some moral imperatives. Control, therefore, becomes the manifestation of the values of a society; a force for the good.

There is also an idea about control as being good in itself; that learning about control, submitting to discipline, makes us better people, and this has been a key principle of a number of different social groups, from religious organisations, to the army, to line-dancing groups. Controlling residents of institutions can, therefore, be presented as giving them skills and abilities which are useful to them. This idea can be found in some child care manuals, where parents are exhorted to encourage self-control in their children, but also in less draconian forms in other types of child care, say where a lack of self-control in behaviour within a residential home is seen as being likely to cause problems for children as they try to develop relationships with others.

The ability to direct oneself, to be disciplined in setting out goals and following strategies, is an ability which is culturally valued, as many of the stories told about successful people illustrate. Stories or myths about great leaders, for example, portray them as determined, focused and strategic, whatever the more precise facts of their biographies might otherwise tell us – indeed, where a 'warts and all' biography does reveal inconsistencies and inaction, we are often disappointed and angry. The value placed on self-discipline, therefore, is inflicted on the most successful in society and the least. Successful figures have to live up to our ideas about self-direction or have their reputations tarnished. The least successful have these values thrust on them and are exhorted to follow these examples and develop these abilities. Those of us in the middle, of course, are free to muddle along, responding to whatever life throws at us.

There are parallels here with the notion of practitioner-centred benevolence outlined above. We control people for their sakes, not for ours. Establishing routines of daily life, restricting certain activities or withholding some resources, the argument goes, teaches service-users the virtues of patience and self-discipline. There is, of course, a more overtly punitive aspect of control, for example in prisons, where the argument goes that the stay here acts as a deterrent against future crimes. If prison is a terrible experience, then people are less likely to act in ways that will mean that they have to repeat the experience. The notion of punitive control, however, is not necessarily confined to institutions which house criminals – a wide range of behaviours can be regarded as undesirable, and anything less than a punitive regime can be seen as encouraging people to indulge in them. This was the case in many institutions in the past, when the catalogue of undesirable behaviour was wider and more rigorously enforced than it is now – homes for 'unmarried mothers' being one example, where regimes were harsh partly in case the women in these homes got the idea that they might get pregnant again. In situations like this, the motives of rehabilitation and retribution become inextricably confused.

For the control of residents to be permissible, whether it is punitive or supposedly therapeutic, service-users have to be defined as lacking in control, and needing some external agency to provide it. This attributed lack of self-control points to some deficiencies of character, awareness or ability in the service-user, and once one deficiency becomes part of the description of a service-user, then it becomes easier to attach more deficits, or to extend the problems already identified. Inability to exercise self-control can be interpreted as a lack of awareness, insight, or social skills, or lack of cognitive or intellectual ability to make decisions or assess situations. This is not to say that identifying the need for control is necessarily a bad thing, without any justification in any circumstances, and there are well-argued and well-supported cases for developing a milieu in which boundaries and expectations are clear for all. Some of the work in therapeutic communities, for example, is about negotiating boundaries and ground rules for behaviour. The problem occurs when control is seen as the sole or primary aim of the institution, with all others subservient to it.

We can appreciate this point more clearly, perhaps, if we consider the attributes and skills that practitioners need in such a situation, where control is paramount. Aside from the purely punitive regime, where presumably practitioners would be advantaged if they showed the sort of enthusiasm for causing suffering which would, in other circumstances, ensure their own incarceration, a regime which is about containment needs people who are consistent in their interpretation and application of the regime. Qualities such as consistency and firmness do not depend on knowledge of anything other than institutional policies, and it is arguable that qualities such as creativity and flexibility are difficult to incorporate into practice alongside them, or indeed are an anathema to them.

Such consistency in the operationalisation of institutional regimes and routines places the practitioner in opposition to the service-user more explicitly than the benevolence model. It is more clear when practice is seen as being primarily about control that the views and preferences of the individual service-user do not count for much, when placed against the institutional view of what should happen. This absolves the practitioners of any obligation that they might feel under the benevolence model to address these preferences – the decisions have already been made, and there is a more open expectation that these would not accord with the views of service-users. Again, if we return to the case of the child who wants to visit a parent, and add to this a set of goals about control rather than benevolence, then the practitioner can simply refer to organisational protocols without having to make any claims about meeting client wishes. Indeed, if practitioners are seen as representatives of the institution, they are placed in opposition to the service-user in immediate questions or disputes, although in the long term they may be portrayed as acting for the ultimate good of the client.

Where practitioners do not see themselves as representatives of the institution, but instead in some other position which is more independent, the conflict then can become between the institution and the practitioner, or between the institution and the client, with the practitioner uncomfortably in the middle. In some circumstances the practitioner may even feel solidarity with the client in his or her struggle with the institution. All of these positions arise where the controlling model of practice becomes rigid and self-validating, in other words where the notion of the institution knowing best becomes the justification for what it does. In this form of argument there is no valid position of opposition – to disagree is to become automatically invalid, because the opposition to the institution's views places the objector immediately in the wrong, as someone who does not have the expertise of the institution. The views of a care worker who argues that the child should visit the parent can be dismissed as ignorant, either about the risks involved or about the importance of control, therefore making an invalid objection.

The paradoxical nature of the 'control for your own good' model, then, gives rise to a number of problems. It devalues the service-user, and ultimately the practitioner, especially if the institution becomes a reified, self-validating entity which cannot be modified or changed by anyone. This process of reification, where the institution becomes regarded as a thing in itself, rather than something which has been created by people and can equally be demolished or changed by them, fits in with notions of practice as control because of the more explicit undemocratic position it takes. Whereas benevolence models may have something to say about the values of the client view and have the client good as an end (however identified as problematic), the control model wipes out the client view right from the start and does not even enter into any debates about the client good. If control is the goal of care, then this can be defined by the institution and circumscribed by it too. The prison system can exemplify this process, where control can be seen as an end in itself, and prisoners released without any thought about what they might do afterwards.

## Practice as enabling

This model of practice owes much to identified deficits in the models discussed above and represents an attempt to move on from them. Essentially, modelling practice as enabling draws on assumptions of benevolence – there is still the idea that practice is about helping people, but the model takes a more critical approach to some of the issues about how the 'good of the client' might be defined. Although it is a move towards the client-centred notion of benevolence that we noted above, it is critical about this rhetoric too. Enabling people is not simply about giving them what they want or ask for (even within resource constraints) but it is also about thinking through the immediate and longer-term impact of such input. With perhaps one ultimate goal being increased client independence, actions and inputs are framed according to the potential they have for increasing this.

The idea of practice as enabling draws on a number of different lines of thought and appears under a number of titles and descriptions. What these discussions take into account, perhaps more explicitly than other debates, are the issues of power in the client and practitioner relationship and, indeed, in the whole structure of care provision. Service-users can be disempowered in many ways, and to different degrees. The position of having a problem, of any sort, and having to rely on others to help is, just in itself, a position which involves a degree of loss of agency – the problem necessitates help, but whether others will give the help that you want, in the way that you want it, or even if they will give help at all is largely outside your control.

Disempowerment is compounded by certain types of problem which provoke certain responses. Problems which are interpreted by others as indicating a lack of ability to make decisions and choices, for example a mental health problem, or even just being a child or an older person, can be met with responses which either explicitly or implicitly dismiss the views of the service-users or any choices that they might express. Problems which are interpreted by others as being self-inflicted, for example anything in the broad definition of 'antisocial behaviour', can evoke a punitive response which is actually validated in the eyes of society if it conflicts with personal choices. To allow these choices is seen as 'pandering' to service-users.

At a broader level, it is argued that service-users come to a service with less power than others because of their marginalisation in society, which takes away access to resources and audiences. This may be because of the characteristics which justify institutional intervention or, more complexly, there may be an interplay between other characteristics, such as race and gender, which can also lead to marginalisation. This relationship is difficult to disentangle, but observations that black people are more likely to be admitted to mental health hospitals raises the question of whether there are a set of pejorative assumptions which lead to this bias in admission, and whether these assumptions also contribute to marginalisation when people are in the institution. This reduced access may well create the problems which necessitate requests for help, so part of this help needs to address this disempowerment if the situation is to move on from a cycle of disadvantage and dependency.

The next chapter explores ideas of power in more depth, as we start to look at the finer details of how practice happens and how models are played out in everyday interactions. For the moment, focusing on a more abstract level of discussion, it is useful to move on from a sketch of what disempowerment might be in order to look at principles of empowering practice and how these translate into views of the service-user, the practitioner and the service. We have already said that the goals of empowering practice are not just about giving service-users a choice and a say in the immediate context of care, but also in developing long-term empowerment, so that service-users can think strategically about the way they use services, what they want from them, and indeed if they want them at all. This last issue, of whether service-users might want to stop using services, sounds like a radical question to ask – we are more used to assuming a need and debating about the detail of how a service can meet it, than asking whether people might want to move out of service use altogether.

At one level, moving away from services can represent one particular ideal goal – the mark of a service that has worked is that users do not need it any more. Examples might be users' groups which are important when people first experience particular problems, say for example a physical illness, but which also become redundant as they help people in the processes of adaptation and adjustment. Adopting this goal indiscriminately, however, may well set up some difficulties and result in entirely inappropriate approaches. Some things do have a limited impact on some people and service-users do adapt to or resolve their problems and move on. Other problems, however, are enduring, and expecting people to move on comes very close to dismissing and discounting their experiences. Nonetheless, services which expect people to remain dependent on them forever, and set up systems which push people into permanent use or discourage moving on, arguably provide a service which does little more than ensure its own continuation.

The enabling model of practice, as with all models, runs the risk of developing service goals which become slogans rather than carefully thought through responses to service-users – enforcing enabling practice, irrespective of differences in individual service-users' circumstances or preferences. This said, the enabling model of practice does carry an idea of the service-user which is positive in comparison with other models. If practice is about enabling the service-user, then the service-user must therefore, according to this argument, have the potential to be enabled. This contrasts with other models which promulgate a view of the service-users which is built around their assumed deficits, be it lack of control, lack of knowledge, frailty or inadequacy.

In the enabling model of practice this positive view of the potential of the service-user to become independent and the awareness of differences in power combine to develop an interest in the service-user as a partner in care. The service-users, then, are actively involved in assessing their needs, reviewing available provision, and making decisions about what they will receive. Indeed, their care is not simply 'received', it is shaped and directed by them. This may involve providing service-users with information, or helping them to locate it, so that they can evaluate their options. It might involve providing service-users with resources, so that they can care for themselves or actively purchase care. At another level it may mean making decision-making processes collaborative and open, with service-users leading the process.

The other side of this partnership is the practitioner, and this role requires different skills to other models of practice. While the general 'kindness' of the practitioner in the benevolence model remains important, other skills are also required, particularly in communication and negotiation with service-users. Practitioners may need facilitation skills to help people find and access resources, or to develop their own. They may need advocacy skills and counselling or advisory skills which are used to help people decide on their options and support them as they pursue these options. These are skills which move beyond 'kindness' yet retain that benevolence, and are focused in the way that practice as control requires, but without the narrowness of aims.

## Summary of the three models

It would be easy to conclude that the practice-as-enabling model is the 'best one', but to do so would be a little too easy and, correspondingly, misleading. While there is a logical force behind this argument which arises from the deficits identified in the other models, if the previous discussion has shown anything, it has shown how complex these models are, and how they overlap and echo each other.

The following table is an attempt to disentangle the models in terms of their key characteristics, as identified in the discussion here. Laying them out like this does help clarify differences and distinctions, but it does so at the expense of portraying the subtlety of these models and the way that they can coexist, intertwine and provide counterpoints to each other.

| Model of practice | Attributes of service-user | Attributes of practitioners |
|---|---|---|
| Practice as benevolence | Dependent, grateful | Kind and well-meaning |
| Practice as control | Lacking in agency | Consistent and firm |
| Practice as enabling | Having potential for independence | Skilled communicator/facilitator |

Nonetheless the table does give us some degree of structure for thinking and analysis, and offers more of a possibility that we can think about practice and identify instances where these models seem to be shaping action. Perhaps then we can make some more open and reflective choices about the way we want practice to go, rather than be caught up in the momentum of a set of ideas that no-one has articulated or challenged.

## Process models of practice

These models, above, are mainly about the goals of practice and how these play out in terms of the desired attributes of practitioners and the assumed attributes of service-users. There are also, however, some models which are more about modes of practice; the ways in which care – benevolent, controlling, enabling or whatever – is delivered. They are not without their own aims but are, in a sense, less explicit than the means by which they are achieved. To clarify the distinction, the models described above can be thought of as emphasising the importance of particular outcomes, whereas models about modes of delivery tend to be presented as being mainly about processes. This distinction is a question of emphasis – process models have outcomes, and outcome models involve processes, but discussions usually focus on one aspect or the other.

Process models, of course, also have implications for service-users and practitioners in the way that they shape the delivery of care. This may not be so explicitly about goals and aims of care, but may have a more immediate and, in the end, more significant impact on care. While models which are mainly about goals tend to be one step removed from everyday practice and the goals may be remote and vague, models which impact on the everyday business of care may well have a more observable and tangible effect.

The range of these models is considerable, and space precludes covering all of them, a task which is made even more daunting as, like the goal-based models, some are implicitly held rather than explicitly stated. We have, therefore, selected some which seem to be key, either because they figure across many debates about care, or because they are recent or current developments in thinking. These seem to fall naturally into pairs of models which oppose each other in fundamental ways, and this is how we have presented them here, as each half of a pair illustrates the other half through the process of opposition. We are aware, however, that in choosing this way to explore these ideas, we may be in danger of setting up irreconcilable differences when, in practice, ideas exist alongside each other, and practitioners move between these seemingly opposing ideas easily and smoothly. Nevertheless, exploring the tensions between the ideas we have identified certainly clarifies them as much by illustrating what they are *not* as much as by outlining what they *are*.

## INDIVIDUALISED CARE VERSUS GROUP APPROACHES

Alongside ways of thinking about service-users as customers (see Chapter 4) are a number of other ideas that are related to, or which follow from, this basic idea. Thinking of the service-users as customers entails some sort of recognition of them as people with preferences and choices that they can exercise. Unless services treat their customers much as Henry Ford is said to have done, when he asserted that his customers could have any colour of car 'as long as it was black', then the notion of customer or consumer means that services have to try to accommodate individual differences in needs and preferences.

There are, of course, other imperatives to treat service-users in ways which acknowledge, and make central to practice, their individuality. These come partly from the disquiet that many felt after examples of non-individualised care were discredited, where every service-user was treated the same, subject to the same routine and provision, where no service-user was allowed to do anything differently to others, or to receive 'special treatment' (or indeed treatment that was in any way a deviation from the norm). While in some contexts and in some periods of history this uniform approach could have been justified as ensuring discipline and the proper subservience in residents, this became less and less tenable as more was realised about the harmful effects of such regimes, and as ideas about individuality as something to be encouraged became widespread throughout society.

Notions of individualised care percolated through all stages of practice. Assessment, for example, became an assessment of the unique needs of each individual, rather than an exercise in categorisation – seeing which label could be applied to the service-user. Planning care followed on from this individualised assessment, as did care delivery, and the evaluation of care necessarily involved the service-user at some point, if only as the original assessment and goals were revisited. Individualised care can involve major and more mundane aspects of care, but it is actually at the mundane level where it can appear most striking. Choosing meals, for example, seems trivial, but the difference between giving everyone the same food, regardless of preference, or giving every individual the opportunity to choose what he or she wants is a clear and graphic illustration of the differences between individualised and non-individualised care.

The main point about individualised care, then, is that it is client centred, rather than organization centred. The difference between assessment and categorisation is illustrative of these two positions and is worth describing more fully. The assessment of a particular service-user might involve asking questions about problems, resources, goals and ideas that the service-user has. This would probably result in some form of outline of what this person's needs are in terms of this unique individual constellation of possibilities and constraints. Organisationally, the service-user might be entered in the records under a category which the organisation uses to map out the client group – for example in health this may be some sort of diagnostic label. People with a range of mental health problems, for example, might be assessed according to the difficulties they are experiencing, the strategies they are using and the resources that they have, and then be entered in the records as 'schizophrenic'.

The difference is stark and obvious: the first is an example of care which is individualised, while the second clearly is not – it flattens out individual differences. It also illustrates differences in the way that practice happens and in the way that this is shaped by different imperatives. The individual assessment is carried out by a practitioner who is involved in planning and delivering care, and so anything other than individualised information does not seem to be very useful. The organisational practices of categorisation, however, are for different reasons – about estimating need and usage at a client group level, and individual preferences do not have much relevance for this.

And yet these distinctions, between assessment and categorisation, which seem so obvious, are distinctions we make on the basis of a particular way of thinking about care, which has not always been prevalent and in some places today is still regarded as slightly eccentric. At different points in time and places of care, practitioners have felt that categorising someone as a schizophrenic told them all they needed to know about what care was needed. Each category had a routine treatment package attached and the planning of this was based on ideas about the general problems that people within this category have, rather than any individual needs. In a sense, what we called an organisational practice above – the crude classification of people for the purposes of general monitoring and planning for a client group – is not always very different from care practice; it can and does sometimes become impossible to distinguish between the two.

That we can do so at all is a reflection of the ways in which we recognise that decisions made about a client group are not parallel with decisions about individuals – that they are different types of decisions. This observation has a logical force to it which seems self-evident, yet the logical argument that what was good for a group would be applicable to its members also has some coherence about it too. That this second argument does not seem tenable anymore is due, as we mentioned above, to the realisation that evidence from practice has clearly demonstrated that while batch processing – giving everyone the same treatment – might work in a car factory, it does not work with people, who are more complex than machines. Serving everyone the same food might be easier for the organisation, but not better for those who have to eat food that they might not like. This is particularly the case when the aims of care shift from, say control and containment, to some idea of therapy with beneficial outcomes for the service-user. Another imperative towards individualised care can be identified in much broader, culture-wide ideas as the importance of individuality is celebrated. While 'fitting in' might be one set of aims that we have, we also pride ourselves on our differences, and this way of thinking, coupled with ideas about benevolent care, leads to the conclusion that care should also take note of individual differences.

Adopting this stance, however, does not in itself make individualised care happen, and the history of institutions indicates that the problems require more thought than simply the adoption of slogans. There are problems, for example, of maintaining a sense of service-users' individuality in institutions, which are about the social context of care and the environments in which it happens. In community care, for example, the opportunities for meeting with clients in their own homes are more common, and this can reinforce identity in a way that meeting in an institution cannot. A visit to a client's home immediately involves stepping into his or her cultural and social milieux, with all its clues to the life that the client lives outside care. The furnishings, the decor and the possessions in the client's home contribute towards understanding the client as a unique individual with particular tastes, preferences and practices. In an institution, these cues are not always so apparent, as the service-user typically has little say about the furnishings and location of the institution. This makes individuality less visible than in the community, and there are other social factors, such as ownership of territory, which are less evident in institutional care. In the client's home, entry is permitted only with the client's permission, and the practitioner is clearly going into the client's territory. In an institution, such ownership is not evident and, if anything, it may be that the client feels a sense of encroaching on the practitioner's ground.

Strategies for maintaining a sense of the client's individuality are various, and range from environmental tactics through to ways of organising staff systems for giving care. Managing the environment to emphasise individuality can involve simple provision of single rooms rather than dormitories to encourage service-users to modify their environment, for example bringing in furniture and possessions as in residential care for older people. Other strategies may involve systems of care and the procedures set out for it, for example the requirement for staff to complete individualised assessments and record these. Yet other strategies involve the organisation of staff through processes of allocation. Approaches such as key worker or primary nursing systems explicitly link up individual clients with individual members of staff and make these individual staff members responsible for negotiating care with the clients – either very formally through assessment and planning, or less formally through responsibilities for the delivery of care. The more formal systems allocate responsibility and accountability for care to members of staff, while in less formal systems care delivery may be overseen by senior staff. Nevertheless, some of the thinking behind such schemes is that the service-users will know who is their member of staff, and the relationship will become more individualised as the practitioner gets to know them as unique people rather than simply one of a crowd.

The success or otherwise of these approaches is, of course, variable and all are prey to difficulties and problems. Environmental strategies are limited by resources, and space and practice strategies such as assessment schedules can simply become paper exercises. Similarly, staff allocation schemes can work to greater or lesser degrees; however, weaker forms can become simply a mechanistic strategy for sharing out workloads and fail, as staff and workloads change, to provide continuity of care.

There are a number of explanations given for these problems and failures of individualising strategies. Menzies (1960), for example, explained the ways in which nurses avoided close contact with patients as being a defence against anxiety generated by dealing with suffering and distress, and there are a whole raft of other explanations available about stress, motivation, workplace cultures and the like. Indeed, in some ways this book could be seen as being largely about developing ideas for taking the notion of individualised care forward. Some of these tensions and problems can be located in the dynamics of relationships between staff and service-users, and the next chapter will discuss these in more detail. At a conceptual level, which is what this chapter is about, there are some problems in the theoretical formulation of care being about individual clients and their needs, when care takes place in an environment which contains a group of clients.

This does not just give rise to a set of pragmatic and logistic problems of balancing the preferences and needs of different individuals within resource constraints, but also suggests that the model of individualised care has serious shortcomings if it cannot accommodate or address issues of caring for groups. A model or framework which focuses exclusively on the staff/client dyad has problems in taking into account other dynamics – the relationships between clients for example, and how this can impact on care.

Models of group care provide a counterpoint to individualised care in the way that they explicitly engage with group dynamics as a factor in care. In this way they add another element to the simplistic view of the alternatives as being between individualised care, which recognises individual differences, and batch processing, which flattens them out. Models of group care acknowledge that care in settings where groups of service-users live together has to address the nature of this living, which is not about separate discrete individuals existing in splendid isolation from each other, but about living in an environment alongside others.

The dynamics of groups and their potential as a therapeutic tool have been explored in a number of ways. Bion (1961), for example, who worked with groups of war veterans after the Second World War, developed the technique of using group rather than individual therapy sessions to explore the traumas that the veterans had suffered. His proposition was that the group dynamics were qualitatively more than simply a collection of individual psychologies. These ideas have been explored through a range of theoretical frameworks, from psychoanalytic theory to systems theory, and have found expression in a range of practice models, from the therapeutic communities in the mental health services to ideas about group living in the care of young people (De Board, 1990). Ideas about group care provide a counterpoint to ideas about the absolute virtues of individualised care. While individualised care may counter some of the worst excesses of batch-processing in institutional care, it is by no means a panacea, and ideas about group care remind us of the limitations of the individualised care model.

## HANDS-ON VERSUS ARM'S-LENGTH

Another pair of practice models which can be contrasted with each other are about forms of care in a very fundamental way. The first model, which is in some respects the one with the longest history in care practice, is the 'hands-on' model, which depicts the business of care as being essentially about meeting with service-users face-to-face and delivering care. This may be physical care, as in professions such as occupational therapy, physiotherapy or nursing, or less observable forms of care, such as counselling, advice and support. Both forms of care which, of course, can be combined, depend on contact between the practitioner and the service-user in an immediate and personal way.

The second model, which could be called the 'arm's-length' model, however, presents practice as something that can be done without any proximity to the client necessary. At its most extreme form there might be no contact at all, with the role of the practitioner being concerned primarily with providing care through intermediaries, with the supervision and direction of other workers and carers. This extreme form seems, expressed this way, to be quite ludicrous; indeed it seems to bear no resemblance to practice at all. It sounds more like some sort of management role, with practice simply being carried out by a different group of workers.

The arm's-length model, however, can be distinguished in a number of recent developments in the care professions, where qualified professional practitioners are increasingly taking on an arm's-length role and unqualified workers drafted in to provide the hands-on care. Developments such as care management in social work and ideas of 'advanced practice' in nursing, which contain a management element, are examples of this move whereby professionals become responsible for the hands-on practice of others, rather than engaging in direct provision themselves.

The care management role incorporates ideas such as brokerage, where services are identified and selected on behalf of the clients or in partnership with them. These services then deliver the immediate care, with the care manager monitoring and evaluating the package of services. What this type of model does is move staff, typically qualified staff, away from direct provision to a supervisory or managerial role. As such, this move can be fostered or encouraged by professional groups as a means of enhancing professional status. Hands-on care is not always valued in our culture, particularly if it involves practice which does not require technical expertise, but simply expertise in communication and understanding. These areas of expertise connect with ideas about 'normal' and 'natural' skills which are innate (particularly in respect of women as 'caregivers') and are, therefore, not prized. Technical skills, such as those of the archetypal brain surgeon, are prized. In a relatively recent development, managerial skills have become valued, as they have been presented as specialised and technical too. The more skills are seen as beyond the everyday realms of common sense or ordinary knowledge, the more they are valued, and part of the impetus towards arm's-length care can be viewed as a consequence of a professional desire to move from low status 'menial' care-giving to higher status managerial roles.

This move also has some financial and organisational imperatives, simply because it is cheaper to have a small number of expensive professionals managing a larger number of cheaper, unqualified staff than it is to have the entire staff group composed of professionals. Euphemisms such as 'skill-mix adjustments' are based on this logic, and skill mix often translates into minimum levels of qualified staff. Organisationally, too, it can be simpler to manage a small number of professionals to manage others, than it is to directly manage a large number of professionals – sometimes the steeper a hierarchy, the less those at the top have to worry about.

On a less cynical note, it is arguable that the type of management that professionals can provide in the supervision of other staff is more appropriate and effective than could be provided by general managers without professional training and experience. It is also arguable that professionals need to broaden their remit to take on board management issues rather than be trapped at the 'care face' with limited impact on the organisations that shape care practice.

Nevertheless, there are many professionals who feel uncomfortable about this move away from direct care, and this can be for a number of reasons. There are, for example, legitimate concerns about the quality of care provided by unqualified staff, and the level of support and training they receive. The paradox is, of course, that if unqualified staff go beyond a certain threshold of training and become equivalent to professionals, then they lose their advantage in cost terms – they are just as expensive.

Perhaps one of the most significant areas of concern expressed is that professionals feel themselves to be no longer practising, just managing. Monitoring others is not seen as care practice – this is, in many practitioners' views, a hands-on activity. Most importantly, the arm's-length model involves only an indirect relationship with service-users, and it is conceivable that there might be no contact at all. If care practice is seen as people work, then moving to an arm's length model makes this people work more and more remote.

## Conclusions

Having visited a number of the models of practice that we have identified (and others may well find different ones), we have tried to demonstrate how we think these ideas impact on practice. They provide a logic and rationale for care, its aims and the form it takes. We have deliberately ended with a debate between hands-on and arm's-length models because this seems to us to be at the heart of debates about care, whether it is a personal activity with a foundation in people skills and communication, or whether it is a more abstract and distanced activity. We would support the argument that care is an interpersonal activity, and find the arm's-length model to be limited in its usefulness for engaging in the debates that need to take place about how care can be developed. The models of management, as we discuss in Chapter 4, come from a general set of theories which are, by and large, about managing anything across the world of industry, and we would argue that there is, or ought to be, a big difference between production lines in factories and care processes, and that this is to do with the extent to which people-centred issues are made focal.

In order to take this idea further, however, we need to explore the interpersonal nature of care in more detail than would be possible in the conclusion of a chapter like this, which has covered a great deal of ground. The next chapter, therefore, takes the time to do this and is intended to look in greater detail at how the statement that care is an interpersonal activity plays out in practice.

# Interpersonal processes   6

## Introduction

The previous chapters have outlined some of the issues and debates which occur around notions of professional practice in institutions. In writing these chapters we took a broad view of institutions, talking about the general nature of the way that work in institutions happens, or is seen to happen. A broad view, however, is not the only perspective that can be taken, and it carries with it some problems in the way that it can shape our analysis. When we think about institutions in this broad sense we often reify them, in other words accord them an independent existence and power outside our control. The 'institution' moves from being a name we give to a type of social grouping or activity to something which has a life of its own. We begin to talk of 'institutionalisation' as if it was something that the institution does, rather than something that the people in it do to, or with, each other. We begin to feel that we are powerless against it, that this process is inevitable. But an institution is a human construction – it is about people, and it is people who shape it.

There are many ways of doing this shaping, and indeed one of the aims of this book is to explore them. What we want to focus on in this chapter, however, is the way in which interpersonal processes, between those who work in institutions and those who live in them, can shape and are shaped by institutional living. The research literature in this area, not surprisingly, deals extensively with the very striking scenarios in which processes are dysfunctional or relationships go wrong, and this literature is important in the way it can show us what to avoid or guard against. There is also some research, however, which has looked at scenarios in which interpersonal processes have been supportive and therapeutic within an institutional context, and this is also important in the way in which it can direct practice in positive ways.

This chapter aims, therefore, to outline the role of interpersonal skills development as a major professional tool at both personal and institutional levels. There are, however, tensions and potentials within the individual and management perspectives which need to be discussed, in other words the way in which individual practice takes place in a particular organisational context. In exploring the significance of the interpersonal exchange between residents, between staff and residents, and between staff, we also explore the relationship of the interpersonal exchange to notions of institutionalism and managerialism.

## Interpersonal processes between residents

We have chosen to begin this discussion with interpersonal processes between residents, primarily because these are not often recognised or given prominence in many texts. This omission, once noticed, becomes quite mysterious as we think about the daily activities of residents in many institutions. While they may interact with staff at specific occasions throughout the day, for therapy, for meals, and for personal care, the people that they are much more likely to spend more time with are other residents. This seems a fairly obvious feature of residential life, but for some reason it does not get seen in the same degree of detail as other relationships or processes in the institution, or accorded the same importance.

If we return to Goffman (1961), for example, we find a cursory and dismissive picture of relationships between 'inmates'. He describes these relationships as transient and instrumental; fleeting alliances between people for mutual gain; and casual *ad hoc* exchanges, which he describes as fraternisation. These relationships belong to the underlife of the institution. Other images of relationships between residents of institutions are presented when Goffman talks of abusive interpersonal processes, bullying and domination, and hierarchical relationships between inmates; power being based on inmates' proximity to staff – the degree to which responsibility is delegated to them. These negative processes also find a place in popular culture – drama and writing about the abuse which inmates suffer or inflict on each other.

Alongside these images of shallow or brutal relationships there are other, perhaps less prominent, ideas about residents supporting each other. Some of these ideas are about residents of institutions coming together in the face of staff brutality or harsh regimes – the story of the orphanage, the prison camp or the army, where inmates find comfort from each other is a common one. What is perhaps less widespread is the story of residents who have relationships in much the same way as other people; positive friendships as opposed to defensive alliances.

Evidence from some ethnographic studies of institutions indicate that these relationships can and do develop. Work in care homes and facilities for older people, for example, suggests that these residents can develop close relationships with each other in which they share experiences, debate issues and discuss choices. Some of these may involve a limited amount of personal disclosure and exchange – what Gutheil (1991), for example, has termed 'companionship'. Other interpersonal processes involve a greater degree of intimacy and can have considerable personal impact. It is tempting, however, to start 'ranking' interpersonal processes as being better or worse according to the degree of intimacy involved. The consequence of this, of course, is that we start to see only intimate relationships as being important, whereas the range of interpersonal processes that people engage in have different ways of being important. The casual exchange with a shopkeeper, for example, cannot be described as intimate, but this does not mean that we would not miss it if it did not happen. It says something to us about the friendliness of the world, the way in which social conventions and habits are played out, and the part we play in maintaining them. The relationship, then, can indicate something about our world and our place in it, as a customer, an independent adult, a social being. Similarly, the fact that exchanges between residents do not involve disclosure of their most intimate personal details does not mean that we can dismiss it as trivial or of no importance.

The problem is, of course, that as members of staff we are not always able to know what happens in these exchanges, or even that they occur. Part of this ignorance may be simply because of the demands on staff time, which reduce opportunities to participate in the social networks of residents, but some of it may also be because we do not have the ability to see these networks when we come across them. If we expect interpersonal processes between residents to be limited to 'fraternisation', then that is what we will see. Again, an example comes from nursing and residential homes for older people. In one study where residents talked at length about their relationships with other residents, staff, when asked about this, denied that these relationships existed, saying that they had not seen it happen (Reed and Payton, 1996). Where residents died, for example, the staff asserted that the other residents were not distressed, or even seemed not to notice. The interviews with the residents, however, indicated that they grieved for their fellow residents and were distressed by the lack of recognition of the death displayed by the staff.

Not seeing these interpersonal processes and not according them any importance stems from ideas about the life of residents, about what sort of people they are and what is important to them. The strangeness of this blindness is more apparent if we try to think about ignoring other relationships in other settings. When we start a new job, for example, we are often asked, 'What are the people like?', because we have ideas that interpersonal processes with colleagues are an important way in which our enjoyment of our job can be shaped. If our colleagues are unfriendly or vindictive, or if we simply do not find them interesting, then work would be less enjoyable than if we spent our days with people that we liked and trusted. Not seeing these interpersonal processes is pretty well unthinkable.

What is happening then, when we do not see the relationships of residents, is that we are thinking of them as somehow being different from ourselves. The justification is a tautology – they are different from us because they are residents, and they are residents because they are different from us. Furthermore, we are not just reflecting a set of assumptions; we are perpetuating them. If we only see what we expect, then the idea that residents' interpersonal processes do not matter becomes a self-fulfilling prophecy. The resident who goes to her room when a friend dies is assumed to be unconcerned rather than mourning, and if we do not actively look for indications that our assumptions are shaky, then we will never challenge them.

There are, however, other ideas about interpersonal processes between residents. These range from the pragmatic view that people in particular situations and with particular problems can usefully share goals and views, to a more extended idea that such sharing is therapeutic. The pragmatic view can be seen in the rise of self-help groups and pressure groups, where people with particular problems come together. Some such groups are primarily about exchanging information about problems – information which might not be accessible or offered to individuals. The value of the group is that members can collate and disseminate information to each other, rather than rely on the vagaries of professional knowledge and willingness to share.

Other groups have developed in other ways. Some provide services, ranging from equipment to personnel; others fund research and development; and others become lobbying groups which campaign for a wider base for service provision and research programmes. The existence of such groups of service-users is a feature of current health and social care provision, and one which is generally welcomed, at least publicly. Such groups suggest that service-users are 'empowered', or at least empowering themselves, and that with the flourishing of consumerism the passive service-users who meekly accepted the services they were given, and the verdicts of professionals about what was best for them, are fast disappearing. While privately, some may have reservations about the ways in which these groups work, and may resent the way in which they can make service delivery more difficult for professionals, in the way that they provide a constant challenge, it is difficult to find a morally acceptable position from which to object – criticisms tend to sound very defensive.

Part of the difficulty lies in the strength of the moral consensus around the notion of power sharing between service-users and providers. The move away from regarding professionals as all-knowing and all-powerful is fuelled by stories of how this knowledge and power can be used to the advantage of professionals rather than service-users. As society becomes more critical of 'expertise' in care, the grounds for arguing that these experts should make decisions becomes less tenable – service-users are making claims to expertise too (personal experience of a problem) and therefore demanding a part in decision-making.

Implicit in this view is the idea that service-users can be thought of as a group, with common interests and goals, and that their collective activity is for mutual benefit. While this position is certainly one that might well be challenged, and it might be thought that there are a number of differences between group members, it does point to the way that we can think of relation-ships between service-users as beneficial and positive, and even something to be encouraged. In user group activity then, we recognise the potential value and legitimacy of interpersonal processes between service-users.

Why, then, do we not recognise the legitimacy of interpersonal processes between service-users when these service-users are residents of institutions? Again, this may stem from the expectations we have of residents, which do not include seeing them as active social beings. Much of the user group activities appear to us through the media, but these images are sometimes difficult to take with us into the workplace. A more explicit way of recognising the importance of interpersonal processes between residents is offered by theoretical positions which have developed these relationships as therapeutic tools. These have taken many forms over the years, ranging from psychodynamic to systemic approaches, but the common factor is the recognition that residents engage in a range of social activities and that these can have an impact on their development.

Some of this work began in contexts where groups of people with shared experiences needed therapy, for example work with soldiers returning from the Second World War. Bion (1961), one of the pioneers of group therapy at this time, developed an approach which was based on the idea that by engaging in group exchanges, these soldiers could have a positive effect on each other. Some of the thinking was pragmatic – there were a lot of soldiers to treat, and not enough resources to provide individual therapy – but there was also some recognition that a group of people were more than the sum of their parts; that 'the group' had its own dynamics which could contribute to the resolution of problems. Interestingly Goffman, in describing group therapy, argues that it could be another way of depersonalising inmates: by forcing them to disclose their feelings in such public arenas, another assault is made on their privacy. This is an important point, that group work can become coercive and antitherapeutic, and again it indicates that techniques alone do not guarantee positive experiences for residents and staff.

Bion's group therapy had roots in Freudian theories and analytic approaches, where personal development comes through exploration of intrapsychic processes. Another approach, which focuses on more social levels of analysis, is systemic therapy, where individuals are seen as being part of a social system in which problems are constructed. Therapy in this approach is directed towards these processes of construction; in a family therapy context attention might be paid, for example, to the processes by which one child becomes identified as 'a problem', while another may not. Systemic approaches pay attention to the dynamics between people in groups, and the stories they create between them. The purpose of this exploration is to develop an awareness of the alternative stories that may be possible.

This book is not about giving instructions about how to use these approaches – there is not enough space here, and other texts are available to do this. These approaches are used here, rather, as examples of ideas that we can have about the interpersonal processes between residents. We do not have to think about them as transient and trivial, but we can think of them as potentially important. This importance can be in the way that relationships offer support, self-validation and a social role, or conversely in the way that they can be destructive. Bullying and intimidation of residents has an impact on residents' lives as much as support and companionship. In being aware of the importance of interpersonal processes then, we would do well to be alert to negative as well as positive dimensions. This alertness, however, depends on being aware of these interpersonal processes in the first place, on developing the ability to see them, and on not simply looking through the lens of the assumptions we make about residents.

## Interpersonal processes between residents and staff

Interpersonal processes between residents and staff have received more attention in research and writing about institutions. It is not very surprising that this is the case, given that the people who read this material are more likely to be staff than residents, and that the people who produce it, who obtain research grants and publishing contracts, are more likely to be members of academic institutions or practitioners than residents of care institutions.

There are, however, other reasons for concentrating on this form of relationship. One is the impact that this can have on residents' lives, because of the differences in power between staff and resident. While relationships between residents are not always equal (residents can exercise power over each other in a variety of different ways), the power that staff can exercise over residents has a different flavour, given the way that it can be sanctioned by the societal processes that lead to the establishment of institutions in the first place. Ideas that residents are incapable of making their own decisions, for example, can serve as a rationale for staff making decisions for them. At a more pragmatic level, the power that staff have to control resources and facilities means that staff have more potential to affect the life of residents in material ways, either adversely by withholding resources or positively by making resources available.

Indeed, one of the themes running through much of the research and debate about interpersonal processes in institutions is that of the power that staff exercise over residents. Power is, however, a more problematic idea than we often assume – we use the term frequently, and do not often spend time unpacking it or scrutinising the meanings that it can have. There are, for example, questions we can ask about the sources of power (who has it and why), and the ways in which it is exercised and the outcomes that it has, and what it does. The picture is made more complicated by the way in which different writers use the term differently, which makes analysis extremely difficult. There is also a point at which it becomes unclear whether the power being talked about is power at an interpersonal level, or at an organisational or societal level. Nevertheless, ideas about power are constantly invoked in the literature, and often usefully so.

### EXPERT POWER

Ideas about power, for example, point us to an examination of how people come to have it (or not have it). For professionals working in institutions, one of the sources of power may be their assumed expertise – a reworking of the saying that 'knowledge is power'. The possession of a distinct body of knowledge is one of the characteristics often attributed to professions. The systems of training that they set up, the processes of examination and registration, and the restrictions placed on people without these qualifications to do certain things, all point to the importance of protecting knowledge from raids by non-professionals. For those outside the profession, then, this knowledge is inaccessible and mysterious – they do not know what it is or, therefore, how it can direct action. This has two consequences: first, it makes the things that professions do seem strange and unpredictable, because action is not based on 'lay logic'; and second, it makes the things that non-professionals do seem dangerous and inept. The rationales for professional action are hidden from view, and unintelligible to the non-professionals in a way which makes their own activities immediately suspect. When confronted with dealing with a situation, it is difficult to act as a professional would and, because we assume that the professional would act in an informed and effective way based on extensive and sound knowledge, the non-professionals cannot aspire to this effectiveness because they do not have this 'insider' knowledge.

This type of 'expert power', then, is derived from the assumptions people make about the nature of professional knowledge. As every professional knows, however, these assumptions would not always be borne out if we actually examined the knowledge we have, for its validity and veracity, or the things that we do, for their basis in this knowledge. Disclosing these weaknesses in our rationales, however, would make us vulnerable – not only would we have to confess to uncertainty, but we might also be challenged or deposed because of our confession. As Freidson (1994) has argued, professionals need to feel decisive – that there is only one course of action to take – because in a climate of 'hot action', where a response is required immediately, debating the options is not possible. This decisiveness, where any action is better than none, is more about the professionals' feelings about themselves than about its impact on the situation. Moreover, the pressure to be decisive, to be in control, sometimes extends to situations which are not, by any stretch of the imagination, 'hot action'. The temptation to be decisive, and to hide the basis of this decisiveness, can extend from emergency action to save lives to tidying out the linen cupboard.

Expert power can also be claimed by people without professional training, on the basis of a different type of expertise – knowing the system. Staff who do not have a professional qualification can, to a certain extent, mimic the professional staff because they have learned from them, or have observed their activities closely, and this mimicry can pass muster if the client group is unclear about who is who in the institution, beyond identifying staff from non-staff. All staff, however, can lay claim to an expert knowledge about how the system works, how the decisions are made, and why things are the way that they are. This expert knowledge can be justified by its historical validity – the staff made these decisions long ago, before the resident came – but more importantly (especially where residents have been there longer than the staff), by reference to its generality: the knowledge is about residents in general, not just about one individual.

## AUTHORITY

In addition to, or instead of, expert power, staff can have power by virtue of their formal position in the organisation, because of the responsibility that comes with their job. Members of staff can be responsible, for example, for making decisions about where residents sleep, what activities they participate in, and what they eat. Their responsibilities can also include making decisions about the future of the residents: when they should leave or whether they should stay. This power is written into their job description, and they will be held accountable for the way in which they exercise it. Senior staff will confer this power on others, a delegation of authority, and will ask others what they have done with it.

Because authority is conferred by position in the organisation, organisational structure is crucial to the way authority is created. A hierarchical structure, for example, distributes authority unevenly – those at the top of the hierarchy have more authority over more important things, while those at the bottom have less authority over less important things. Crucially, organisational structure places different members of staff in different positions, but also places residents and staff in different positions, most commonly conferring little or no authority on residents. While staff may, on occasion, delegate authority to residents for organising various aspects of daily life, this authority can be taken away at any minute – it is not part of the resident's position, simply something that is given on a personal basis, and can be taken away just as easily.

Authority is a form of power which quite neatly illustrates some of the paradoxes in institutional life. Authority is vested in individuals and organisations by virtue of position, rather than merit. Similarly, the authority vested in institutions often comes from their position in the social world, rather than by merit. With both forms of authority, a closer examination of its justification reveals it to be fairly tenuous, relying on a social consensus as much as anything else. The consensus that staff have authority, that institutions are where authority rests, is rarely challenged, however, so this authority continues to be accepted and exerted.

## PERSONAL POWER

Expert power and authority are types of power which are, to a certain degree, impersonal, that is they can be attached to anyone who has a certain job, or has completed a certain course. The nature of the individuals, their personality or characteristics, is not as important as their formal attributes. Personal power, however, arises from the nature of the individual and transcends qualifications and roles.

Some ways in which personal power operates may be simply a part of the way in which an individual has come to operate in the world, a way which is not premeditated or thought through. Other ways of operating, however, may be learnt or developed. When we talk about interpersonal skills we make this more explicit – the notion of skills carries with it ideas of learning and development. This gives us an option of trying to find ways of developing different forms of personal power or interpersonal skills.

## INTERPERSONAL SKILLS

The discussion of power above sets up some of the considerations which must be part of any discussion of interpersonal processes between staff and residents. It is, however, a negative picture that is painted which indicates that power is 'a bad thing'. Things are not, of course, as simple as that and there are aspects of power, such as the setting of boundaries, which can be seen as therapeutic. This, however, leads us to another point: we do not just have an idea that the interpersonal processes between staff and residents should not be damaging, but we also have the idea that they should be actively beneficial – they should be therapeutic. This positive formulation of interpersonal processes finds expression in a number of ethical positions about the way in which staff should think about those for whom they provide care. Put simply, these ideas are centred on the view that staff should see residents as unique individuals, rather than depersonalised work-objects.

The process of depersonalisation has been described by several authors, and a common picture is that staff begin to see residents not as people but as 'work-objects', in other words things that they do work to, very much as they would regard inanimate objects on a factory production line. Clarke (1978), for example, described unqualified staff working in a hospital ward who moved between this employment and working in local factories, without making much distinction between the two environments. The emphasis in their descriptions of both environments was on 'getting through the work' – in the hospital, work was patient care. They would, thus, see the measure of their work as the speed with which they had completed tasks (such as bathing patients or assembling units in the factory) or the number of such tasks they had completed. Jones (1979) describes the process thus:

> Just as the economies of mass production in the modern car industry are obtained by means of a process of standardisation in which all the cars produced are identical, with parts fully interchangeable between them, so human beings in the barracks style institution were assumed to be identical. (p. 9)

This 'industrial model' of care, of course, carries similarly industrial formulations of goals and aims, namely the efficient and rapid completion of tasks. In such a model, then, individuality becomes an obstacle to work rather than a driving force behind it, and starts to look very much akin to ideas that residents of institutions should have no choices which might interfere with the organisational goals.

A different approach to depersonalisation is taken by Menzies (1960) in her exploration of nursing work. Coming from a psychoanalytic perspective,

Menzies argued that nurses organised their work in such a way that they 'fragmented the patient', as a way of coping with the anxieties engendered by contact with people in pain or who were dying. Organising work so that each nurse was responsible for carrying out one task with all patients (such as bathing, feeding, or medication), rather than all tasks with one patient, was a way of avoiding confrontation with or recognition of the patient as a whole human being. Such recognition would also involve recognition of the tragedy of each patient and result in catastrophic anxiety for staff.

Menzies' description approaches the staff–resident relationship from a particular perspective which views practice as arising from intrapsychic and innate features of the way in which we deal with anxiety and ideas of pain and death. As such the message is, on first examination, a pessimistic one – this is the way that people are. Menzies, however, does indicate that these responses may be modified, or at least ameliorated, if staff are supported in their encounters with residents. The details of what form this support may take are hazy, but at least an argument is being made that such responses are not inevitable. Some of the other descriptions of relationship dynamics are, however, more fatalistic – Goffman's descriptions of stigma, for example, portray this process as if it were as much a feature of human life as the laws of physics. In some ways, however, we should not expect Goffman to provide us with ways out of these dynamics – that is our responsibility. What we can take from this work, therefore, is an awareness of the ways in which our relationships with residents may be shaped, the social and cultural context in which they are developed, and the consequences they can have for ourselves and residents. This awareness can provide a foundation for developing positive relationships. There is another type of discussion which takes in ways of thinking about interpersonal processes as areas of skilled practice rather than culturally and socially determined phenomena which we can accept only as destructive or demeaning.

These discussions are about ways in which staff can develop their practice in a therapeutic manner – the idea here is that staff do not have to accept their responses to residents and ways of working with them as inevitable. The argument is that staff can do something about them. The notion of 'emotional labour', for example, indicates that staff can and do manage their feelings and responses. The term comes originally from work by Hochschild (1983), who studied air hostesses and the way that they coped with passengers, who could sometimes be difficult or even offensive. Surface work involved managing irritation to the extent that hostesses could get through exchanges while remaining pleasant and calm, while deeper emotional labour involved more extensive work. Hostesses would construct a range of different explanations for abusive behaviour, such as anxiety, which meant that they not only tolerated bad behaviour but came to feel some sympathy for those who displayed it.

These ideas of emotional labour have been applied to nursing and the way that nurses manage interpersonal processes with patients. Smith (1992), for example, found that nurses could engage in this 'reconstruction' of the patient, but it was a practice that was learned and developed over time, with novice nurses being less adept than more experienced ones. This learning, however, was affected by the practice environment: when this was supportive, and nurses had role models to follow, students became confident in their ability to engage with patients at an emotional level. Where the practice environment was unsupportive, however, where students were discouraged from talking to patients and where no other staff appeared to value this, they remained uncomfortable with personal discussions and tended to prefer an impersonal approach to their work.

What Smith's work points to is that the response of staff to residents is something that can be 'managed'. The notion of managing interpersonal processes, however, does not sit easily with other ideas about how relationships ought to be spontaneous and natural – if they are not, then they are regarded as manipulative and insincere. The value placed on unmanaged relationships and the accompanying ideas of rapport and compatibility link up with ideas that we have about truthfulness in relationships, that one necessary feature of a 'good' relationship is trust. If we do not have this truthfulness, if we do not react without thought and calculation, then we cannot have trust.

At the same time, however, we have ideas about 'good' relationships which centre on characteristics such as sensitivity and respect. Here the model is about negotiating interpersonal processes so that responses and exchanges are positive, timely, and maintain personal integrity. The sensitive relationship is about placing an emphasis, not on truth alone, but on intention – we support self-control and strategic thinking if the intention is to help, rather than harm.

One area in which self-control, rather than spontaneity, is approved is when dealing with 'difficult' clients or service-users, who are not cooperative or appreciative. A spontaneous reaction, say of disgust or anger, would be regarded as unprofessional and harmful, and so there is recognition of the value of some control of immediate responses. The idea of 'unpopularity', however, is a problematic one, which perhaps can tell us more about ourselves than about service-users. A review of the literature on unpopular hospital patients by Kelly and May (1982) found that much of this work had tried to identify characteristics which 'made' patients unpopular. Some studies had linked unpopularity with age, gender or health problem, but this was not consistent across studies. Kelly and May suggest that it may be more useful to move from trying to locate sources of unpopularity in patients, to thinking of it as something that happens between staff and patients. Their argument is that professionals develop a set of ideas about the way in which a 'good' member of their profession should be; ideas developed from general cultural images, peer group expectations and their interactions with patients. The way in which they evaluate their ability as professionals, therefore, is based on these ideas. If one of the desired characteristics is about being appreciated by patients, then patients who do not appreciate them will make the professionals feel bad about themselves, and uncomfortable around the patient. In other words, what Kelly and May are arguing is that professionals like clients who like them.

This observation, truism though it may seem, takes away from considering the staff–resident relationship as a simple dyad, driven primarily by the personal characteristics of those involved, and moves towards thinking of the relationship as something which takes place in and is shaped by a social world in which values and expectations come into play. With this analysis, then, the way in which the staff approach interpersonal processes with residents stems from the values of their peers and wider society. If a 'good' staff member is thought of, say, as someone who maintains 'discipline', then their interactions and the goals of their interactions will be concerned with ensuring order and regularity, of not allowing individual differences in residents to interfere with the efficient carrying out of routines. If a 'good' staff member is seen as one who is warm and empathetic, and who respects the individuality of residents, then a very different set of interactions and goals come into play.

This is not to say that staff behaviour is a product of 'group think' and that individual differences in approaches and ideas do not make for differences in behaviour. The literature is, as we have earlier demonstrated, full of individuals who took a very different stance to that of their peers; who thought and acted differently to others. These individuals, however, stand out because of the strength of their convictions, and without this it is not easy to behave in ways contrary to peer group norms. Baker (1978), for example, observed a hospital ward in which the ward sister attempted to develop individualised care. This meant abandoning routines, and allowing patients to get up in the mornings, wash, dress and eat when they wanted to, rather than when working practices dictated. This was not approved by all of the other staff on the wards or by managers and senior staff, and when the ward sister was off duty, the other staff reverted back to the usual routinised care under pressure and disapproval, particularly from medical staff.

In conclusion, then, what we are arguing here is that interpersonal processes between staff and residents are not just about the individuals concerned, but about the social world and professional culture in which they happen (for a fuller discussion see Shotter, 1993). It is important also to note here that this social world has many imbalances of power that can shape these processes in very direct ways. There is, for example, literature on race and gender issues which suggests that the way in which relationships in institutions play out can be affected directly by these wider inequalities (McNay, 1992). Black people, for example, are over-represented in psychiatric hospitals, and the argument is that this is not necessarily because they are more prone to mental health problems (although lifelong experiences of racism can contribute to stress and distress), but that society deals with some behaviour of black people with an institutional response (Parker et al., 1995). Coming into a psychiatric hospital, then, is in itself a manifestation of power imbalances in society. There is a further argument that suggests that racism can be continued beyond the process of admission; that black people in institutions suffer from racist attitudes and practices in a number of ways.

Issues of race and gender can, however, also transcend the staff–resident boundaries: in other words, if you belong to a group which is disadvantaged, then this disadvantage permeates your life in whatever you do. There is, for example, a body of work which suggests that staff who are black are promoted less than other workers, and that they are largely employed at unqualified grades. There is also a feminist argument that care work in general is undervalued as 'women's work' and seen as unskilled and unimportant (Doyal, 1983). This has implications for the training and support of staff, which can be deemed unnecessary for such 'natural' work (Aymer, 1992). Wider social contexts and particularly imbalances in power, therefore, can impinge in a number of ways on interpersonal processes in care settings.

An overview of the possibilities for relationships between staff and residents indicates that warm, supportive relationships which respect individuality and contribute to personal development can happen. The idea of interpersonal skills, that staff can develop the ability to form this sort of relationship, contains the idea that they are not necessarily spontaneous and that they can be strategically initiated and developed. Developing these skills, however, is not simply about learning a set of techniques and procedures, because using them will depend on a wider set of issues than personal values, goals and attributes – it will depend on whether using them is permitted, approved or supported within the workplace (Smith, 1992). It is with this in mind that we turn to the next section, in which we debate the dynamics of interpersonal processes between staff: the way in which they can support each other, or the way in which they can constrain each other.

## Interpersonal processes between staff

The discussion of interpersonal processes between residents sketched in some of the dynamics that may exist between them, as a group who live with each other and may have similar needs. This is not to say that residents are all alike, and when we consider another group who have similar interests – the staff – such a view becomes even less tenable. As members of staff, we feel uncomfortable, perhaps even angry, with the idea that we are all the same, yet to an onlooker we perhaps look very much like each other. We share training and educational characteristics, engage in very similar activities, and may even wear a common uniform, whether it be official or informal.

As members of staff, however, we would argue that these features are superficial, and that they disguise great differences. Indeed, as Hugman (1991) has pointed out, it is a mistake to assume that occupational groups are homogenous – there are tensions within groups as well as between them. For members of an occupational group working closely together though, ways have to be found of managing these tensions, otherwise the whole enterprise collapses and loses direction.

When institutional living goes wrong to the extent that a public inquiry takes place, the interpersonal processes between staff are often a central focus of investigation. In the inquiry report we read that there was 'a lack of leadership' or 'low morale'. Recommendations are made about changing management styles or, more often, managers. Part of this emphasis comes from a recognition, albeit covert, that while staff may be in a minority in an institution, the balance of power is such that their impact on the quality of life of residents is not related to their numbers alone.

Another point which is being reflected in the wording of inquiries, and other discussions about institutions, is that there is a balance of power within staff groups. Notions of 'leadership', for example, are related to ideas about differences in influence and role between staff – that they are not all the same. The idea of difference is also built into much managerial literature, especially that aimed at managers, where part of the story told is about the vital difference a 'good' manager can make. There are discussions about motivating other staff, about empowering them and fostering their creativity, in the benevolent literature. There are discussions about monitoring and disciplining staff and about making their work more productive in the rationalist literature. It seems as if, whether the relationship between manager and staff is conceived of as supportive or restrictive, it is still based on differences in power and role.

There is some literature on more egalitarian systems, where no one individual is 'in charge' and where power and responsibility are shared. Staff may be different in their skills and abilities, but the work that they do is not differently valued. Such organisations are rare, however, and a number of reasons can be identified for this. First, institutions develop within a context which is based on hierarchical assumptions. An individual agency or facility is linked into a range of different systems to a greater or lesser extent, for example social or health services, and this system will have established ways of working and communicating which rely on the idea of people being 'in charge'. If no-one is in charge, the other parts of the system have difficulty in relating to it.

Second, there are professionally derived notions of how people should relate to each other in institutions. These are sometimes about how different groups should work together, with professionals engaging in debates about interdisciplinary and multidisciplinary working. There are tensions between recognising the limits of our own profession and the strengths of others, and moving into a position where professional boundaries cease to exist: where staff can become de-skilled workers, crossing boundaries and losing identities. Professions have an interest in maintaining boundaries and identities and not blurring these too much, in order that distinct areas of practice can be retained and recognised, and this imperative can impact on the relationships that staff have with each other. Stories of interprofessional rivalry, with different professions disagreeing with treatment approaches, or about who has the authority to make decisions, are common.

Another set of divisions which originate in professional concerns about power are about the interpersonal processes between qualified and unqualified staff. Again this is concerned with who has authority to make decisions about care, and also about the relative differences in skills that the two groups are assumed to have. These differences, which may be relatively easy to identify in other areas of work, are quite difficult to spot in care work, where much of the practice is dependent on personal qualities and experience. This renders the notion of skill acquired primarily through professional training difficult. Although such training may give people a specific degree and type of knowledge, the question of how they use it still remains. It is possible to identify staff who appear skilled and effective who have not had formal training and, conversely, professionally trained staff who are incompetent. With such ambiguities, there are imperatives to protect the professional status by establishing clear lines between qualified and unqualified staff, which can lead to a range of problems in their relationships and the way that they work, with unqualified staff feeling devalued and restricted in their practice.

This discussion of the divisions between staff, and the possible problems of interpersonal processes, links with notions of organisation and management discussed in more detail in Chapter 4. The key issue for this chapter is about what sort of interpersonal processes we think would be ideal in institutions. If we hold to the idea that the best form of relationship is an open, egalitarian and mutually supportive one, then this pushes us to consider ways of overcoming divisions and hierarchical structures. If, however, we incline to the view that interpersonal processes between staff should be functional, in that they should lead to greater efficiency and effectiveness at work, then there is no necessary problem with hierarchical structures. Indeed, there is an argument that they can be more efficient because everyone has a distinct role and line of accountability.

We can, however, make an argument that interpersonal processes between staff are not simply functional, but they are about creating an ethos or culture within an institution which is open and supportive. Rigid hierarchical systems may do more than oppress the staff – they may well place service-users in the hierarchy and in detrimental positions. While some institutions, for example a large hotel, have rigid and efficient hierarchies which place the service-user, the hotel guest, at the top, in different institutions there are examples of service-users being located very firmly at the bottom of the hierarchy. Rigid role demarcation, then, is not necessarily to the detriment of service-users, but there is always the possibility that it could be.

The notion of open and supportive interpersonal processes between staff seems, on surface examination, to be more likely to offer a positive pay-off to the service-user, in that the ethos that is created is more able to be responsive to needs and preferences. Cosy relationships between staff, however, are not automatically beneficial to service-users – especially if these relationships are exclusive of service-users. Staff supporting each other is one thing, but when it becomes a matter of supporting each other against the clients, then that is a very different matter. Notions of solidarity among staff can become problematic unless this solidarity is extended to include service-users, and avoids identifying them as the people whom it is important to be solid against. Close staff relationships can result in yet another reworking of the 'us and them' theme, with 'them' in this case not being other professionals, other organisations or other grades of staff, but the service-users who should be the centre of the institution.

## Conclusions

This chapter has discussed the complexities of interpersonal processes in institutions, looking at interpersonal processes between service-users, between service-users and staff, and between staff. Of these three areas, the interpersonal processes between clients and staff have received the most attention: there is a huge range of texts which explore the possibilities of therapeutic relationships and the strategies and skills that they require. These texts, however, centre mostly on the staff–client relationship to the exclusion of other interpersonal processes happening in the environment of care. Furthermore, they often explore it only as a relationship between two individuals, rather than look at the wider contexts of staff–client interpersonal processes as interaction between groups of people.

In this chapter, therefore, we have explored interpersonal processes beyond this useful but narrow focus. We chose to begin with interpersonal processes between service-users because this was neglected and under-theorised in the literature. This neglect fails to engage with what can be the most important dimension of institutional life for the service-user – the relationships with others in similar situations, and with whom the client is likely to spend a considerable amount of time. Addressing these relationships, however, moves the practitioners from centre stage, and raises questions about what it is that they offer to clients.

Similarly, we have ended this chapter with some discussion of inter-personal processes between staff, partly as a way of challenging the idea that staff are a homogenous group with shared goals and values. Addressing the differences between staff, and making some decisions about how we want them to work together, seems to be an important step if we are to move away from the simplistic notion of the staff–client dyad as the foundation of care.

In writing this chapter we have, paradoxically, made much use of the terms 'staff' or 'service-user' to stand for groups of people. In so doing, we are aware that we have perpetuated the notion of homogeneity in these groups, while at the same time trying to establish the possible differences within them. In particular, we have perpetuated the notion of difference between these groups simply by the terms we have used, and ironically it is these assumptions of difference that we have challenged elsewhere in the book. Therefore we might argue that we should not keep thinking about people in institutions as staff or clients, but simply as people who share an environment, although for different reasons. It is, however, these different reasons which make all the difference to expectations, attitudes and behaviours. To ignore them would be naïve and dismissive of the pathways that people take to institutions and the experiences that they have there. We have to argue, therefore, that there is a difference between staff and service-users, and we have to engage with this before we can think about whether the differences that we identify or construct are useful or not, and how we might go about moving away from divisions that have no benefit to the central purpose of the institution.

# Values, ethics and practice

**7**

## Introduction

In calling this chapter 'Values, ethics and practice', we wanted to make explicit some of the debates about institutional care that we feel are often brushed over in practice and policy debates. Debates about 'good' care, for example, draw on a range of ethical debates in an implicit way, by referring to hallmarks of good practice which have a basis in debates in moral philosophy. This brushing over is not necessarily a deliberate strategy to mislead – it is difficult to imagine how disguising ethical roots would be seen as advantageous, since we more often see people claiming rather than disclaiming the moral high ground. It is more a matter of the debates being forgotten or misplaced: as earnestly debated principles become orthodox views, and then further degenerate into slogans, the complexities of the issues become lost; ideas are presented as unproblematic when it was, and still is, possible to make a counter-case.

Unpacking the history of these issues can give us some ways of critically examining the slogans that are used in debates about care. There is perhaps a more fundamental issue that could also do with some examination, and that is whether it is helpful or appropriate to think of care as being a moral enterprise anyway. This idea conjures up at least two potential problems. First, by describing care as a moral endeavour, we seem to be suggesting some sort of alliance or connection with other moral agencies, for example a number of religious movements and groups. The activities of these groups are explicitly moral and spiritual and engagement is, by and large, a deeply personal and private one. There are some immediate concerns, therefore, about territory – are we in danger of claiming a territory to which we have no rights? While religious groups may claim this territory because of their stated goals, and the knowledge and expertise that they have, services outside these parameters are generally regarded as secular. Morality is, perhaps, none of our business.

The second, related, concern is that not only is morality none of our business, but to have an explicit moral stance is actively wrong. Memories and tales of institutions of 'moral correction', where residents were subject to privations because of their perceived moral failings, still cast long shadows. Homes for unmarried mothers, for example, seemed to be less about care than correction, with resulting misery. The language of the old psychiatric hospital, with expressions such as 'moral defectives' and the ill-treatment that this seemed to excuse under the guise of discipline, is another example. The spectre of 'moral judgements' built into the *modus operandi* of an organisation is a worrying one.

Yet to think of the institution as completely without any values is seriously misleading. Values are inherent in all human activities, and the development and maintenance of an institution is no exception. The question is, rather, whether these values are moral or not. There are other types of values that might well come into play, such as pragmatic values about efficiency, or fiscal values about cost. These types of values, however, exist alongside moral judgements rather than replace them. Concerns about what is the cheapest way to provide care do not usually prevail entirely, without anyone asking about what the quality of such care might be if costs are reduced too much. After all, the cheapest form of care is no care at all, and the fact that a society is making some attempt to provide care is an indication of reference to another kind of value beyond simply economic concerns.

If we accept this argument, that the creation of services entails some moral or ethical considerations, then we need to look at what these considerations may be, and also to look at how they may have changed or developed over time. Given the long history of many institutions, it seems unlikely that the values of the founders are still held with tenacity by their successors. The first chapters of this book sketched out some of the historical threads running through institutions, and from this history it is clear that ideas about what an institution exists for have changed over time, or have sometimes existed alongside each other. Institutions have been driven by many ideas – of reward, of containment, of sanctuary and of correction – and how these ideas have developed in the past can sometimes explain how things are done in the present.

If we accept the idea of care provision as a moral enterprise, in that it is shaped by some moral and ethical concerns, we can then start to develop criteria for evaluating it which arise from these concerns. The thought of being judged on the ethical basis of the care we give, however, sounds a daunting and even oppressive process. Morals and ethical standards have come to be thought of as very private and personal things in an increasingly diverse and secular society. Where we once might have subscribed to a common set of public values, derived from state or church, for example, morality has become a much more individual thing, with people building up their own sets of values. These individual sets of values are not, of course, absolutely different from each other and exhibit differences in the fine detail rather than broad principles – most people would subscribe to the view that inflicting pain on others is wrong, but some might excuse it under specific circumstances.

Nevertheless, these fine details and interpretations are often jealously guarded, with part of their virtue coming from the idea that they are 'personal'. When we start to talk about some sort of ethical examination of practice, then, we should be on the alert.

This apparent breach of the distinction between personal morality and public activity is, however, not particularly problematic if we start to think of these things as fundamentally connected. Having a personal set of ethics is of limited importance if these values do not shape behaviour in any way, and if someone argued that they thought one thing but did another, they would be met with accusations of hypocrisy or weakness (Midgley, 1981; Olafson, 1973). At this level, then, the idea of public expression of inner values is expected.

Where there is a difficulty, however, is where personal values are incompatible with public behaviour. Where personal values are compromised by the constraints of organisational practices, we tend to think of this as particularly problematic. The problem, however, is more obvious where we think of personal ethics as 'good' and the ethics of the organisation as 'bad'. This is a more common formulation than it was, say, a century ago, where one of the purposes of many institutions was to inculcate more moral behaviour in those who lived or worked in them. The idea of the institution as oppressor and violator of personal morals is, perhaps, more common nowadays.

If we turn this around, however, and return to an earlier notion of the institution as a moral force for good, we have a formulation where the individual is seen as potentially 'bad' and the institution is potentially 'good'. In other words, the impulses and motives of an individual in an institution are not necessarily seen as benevolent, and the practices and systems of regulation in the institutions are held to impose some constraints on the full and frank expression of malevolence. This does not feel so problematic, and in examples where members of staff have been abusive to residents, such regulation and imposition of constraints are exactly what we call for.

The suspicions that we might have about institutional ethics, however, are also about their sincerity. 'Corporate ethics' conjures up images of glossy company brochures and public relations exercises. While personal ethics are viewed as being deeply held, by virtue of their 'personal-ness' it is difficult to think of an organisation going through the experiences and dilemmas and personal reflection that go to make up our individual values. We therefore have suspicions that any claims that an organisation makes to uphold a set of principles is done more as a strategy to increase public acceptance of the organisation than to genuinely promote a moral stance.

At the same time, however, we do feel comfortable about some collective values, for example political principles. While we may not agree with certain political values, we do not necessarily dismiss them as meaningless, because they are not individual but shared. At an even more macro level, we feel comfortable with ideas such as democracy and all of the principles that it entails, such as personal freedom, universal suffrage, or public accountability. Perhaps it is this 'meta-ethic' of freedom that is the key here – while political parties may develop a set of ideas about how society should be organised, we are free to agree or disagree with these proposals, and if we do not have this freedom then we start to feel very worried.

These issues and debates are extremely complex and display a number of tensions. There is the privileging of personal values over institutional ones, not because of the merit of these personal values in terms of their content, but in terms of the processes by which we arrive at them. Personal reflection and experience, no matter how limited, is held to be a better process than any that an organisation could go through. This merit system, however, is bedded into a 'meta-ethic' which values freedom over other things. It is arguable that this ranking is relatively recent – at other times notions of duty and obedience have been more powerful. This is an important point, in case we start to think of freedom as some sort of eternal and universal ethic – it is perhaps as socially constructed as anything else.

Nevertheless, if we accept the importance of the notion of 'freedom' in the way that we think and talk about values today, then this leads us to think through how this freedom can be promoted. In the remit of this book, that involves looking at how the relationship between the values of the individual can be connected to the values that the institution manifests in its structures and practices. This is not only about 'connection' in the sense of correlation (that individual values should match up to the institution, as perhaps we might have thought about it a century ago), but about how the values of the individual can contribute to the development of institutional values, and how this can be enhanced by the way that both individual and institutional values can be articulated and debated. In order to support this process, therefore, the next section explores some possible frameworks for doing this.

## Ethical theories and frameworks: values and principles

Most textbooks on professional ethics will include, at some point, an outline of major ethical theories or frameworks. These frameworks can be classified in a number of ways, for example orientated towards ends (teleological theories) or concerned with processes or means. In other words, different theories place an emphasis on either means or ends as being the crucial determinant of whether an action is ethical or not. In a treatment programme, for example, an ends-based framework would look at the outcome, i.e. whether the treatment worked or not, as being more important than the process by which this result was achieved. A more process-orientated framework would look at the way in which the treatment was delivered as a way of determining the ethical status of an intervention, and would not be so concerned with the outcome. A slightly different way of categorising ethical theories is to talk of them as concerned with duties which lead to actions rather than the good to be achieved by actions – a slightly different formulation of the 'ends versus means' difference. In formal ethical theory, the terms 'deontological' and 'consequentialist' theories are often used to denote this range although, of course, most ethical positions that people take involve elements of both sets of principles.

In this description, deontological theories concentrate on the rightness or wrongness of actions irrespective of their outcome. A key philosopher in this area was Kant (Paton, 1948), who came up with the famous imperative, 'Act only on that maxim whilst thou canst at the same time will that it should become a universal law'. In other words, Kant argued that one way of judging an activity would be to think through what would happen if it was a universal way of behaving. If disaster and confusion would result, then this would not be an adequate moral principle. This excludes activities such as lying which, were it universal, would result in complete chaos, but does point us towards principles such as respecting persons. If such principles can be adopted universally, then the merit of actions can be judged by looking at the way in which they conform to these principles. Appreciation of these principles leads to dutiful behaviour, which is not dependent on special circumstances, inclination or personal preference.

Perhaps the most well-known consequentalist or ends-based theory is the utilitarianism of both Mill and Bentham (Warnock, 1962). Here, actions are judged by their consequences and, more specifically, by the degree to which they maximise the sum total of human happiness. Utilitarianism, therefore, developed detailed formulations of how this happiness might be calculated, and so using utilitarian theories involved trying to work out, for example, whether the extreme pleasure of one person might outweigh the minor discomforts of everyone else. Conversely, there might be a judgement to be made about whether the extreme unhappiness of a few people is a price worth paying for the comfort of the majority. Aside from these calculations, another problem with utilitarian theories is that they are difficult to use in an uncertain world, where outcomes cannot be predicted easily. While they might be useful in evaluating past actions where the consequences are apparent, predicting effects of actions is an extremely difficult business.

A lengthy discussion of ethical theory would be out of place here – there are many other texts which will do this (see Frazer et al., 1992 for an overview and critique of some of these). It might, however, be useful to work through how these ideas might connect up with practice. An example of a duty-based principle might be found in the sorts of professional codes of conduct which set out the standards which professionals seek to follow. These might involve things such as observing confidentiality, acting in the best interests of clients, doing them no harm and the like. More precise codes of practice might deal with the sort of service that the professional should provide and the client should expect, for example frequency of contact, scope of assessment, or method of care delivery. A more utilitarian emphasis may well be found in mission statements and their like, where statements are made about the general purposes of the service and its goals for the client population.

These broad ethical theories serve as a background to some of the issues which are identified in debates about values in care. While these debates may pick up on specific issues, it is often with these theories as points of referral. Sometimes we are exhorted to support certain values on deontological grounds, universal principles, say of rights or freedom, and sometimes on utilitarian grounds of increasing happiness. While some of these key concepts or issues draw upon and stem from a wide range of philosophical debates, about politics and personhood for example, identifying the ethical theories that they refer to, however obliquely, can sometimes provide a useful way of thinking about the positions proposed.

## Key concepts

Throughout the debates on the ethics of care a number of ideas keep cropping up. Sometimes they appear as clusters, terms being tied together or used interchangeably. In many discussions they are placed alongside opposing ideas and the contrasts identified are used to illuminate both. This is often a useful way of exploring ideas and one that we have broadly adopted here, although this approach is not without its problems – sometimes polarities can be artificially created by debate and often the grey areas in between, which are often the most interesting, are neglected. Bearing this in mind then, the following discussions should be taken as covering a range of positions, rather than trying to establish absolute divisions between them.

### EMPOWERMENT AND PATERNALISM

The concept of 'empowerment' is one that is coming dangerously close to degenerating into a slogan, rather than representing a coherent body of values. It is used in a wide range of contexts and situations, sometimes in ways that seem contradictory or incoherent. A central idea behind the use of the word can, however, be traced and this is that service-users are people who tend to exercise less power than others around them, for a variety of reasons (Witz, 1992). The reasons may be because the way that services are organised excludes them from decision-making or the control of resources. Furthermore, this may be because this group is generally excluded from exercising power outside services, through processes of marginalisation. (The complexities of discussions and definitions of power have been outlined in Chapter 6.) This imbalance in power is seen as something to be redressed, for a range of practical and ethical reasons. Practical reasons may take the form of rational justifications for empowerment – the system is ineffective with existing imbalances, and sharing of power can translate into a sharing of responsibilities and a reduction in organisational workload. In some instances, maintaining and exercising power is time consuming and it would simply be easier if service providers did not have to do it.

The ethical rationales are often based on notions of 'rights': that human beings should be accorded the power to shape their lives because they are human beings (Dworkin, 1978). Philosophically, the idea of rights has a long history and stems from political debates about governance. Notions of 'meritocracies', whereby those with most merit, be it principles or skills, govern others, have been proposed in one form or the other, often as an antithesis to monarchies. The process by which this happens, however, is by no means un-negotiated – the idea of a social contract between ruler and ruled is something which recurs in a number of forms and is, at a basic level, that the ruled surrender rights to rulers in exchange for benefits (Rousseau, 1968). What rights and what benefits are involved varies in different formulations, but the principle holds firm that if there is a breach of contract, especially by the ruler, then the contract can be declared void, and the ruled are justified in rebelling against the ruler (Sabine, 1973).

This is, of course, a macro view of rights, but it has some interesting connections with some of the debates we have about rights in care. Ideas that service-users should surrender their rights (to make certain decisions, to do certain things) in exchange for the benefits of being ruled, which may be described as rational guidance, protection 'against themselves' or simply care, are fairly explicit in, say, Victorian literature on institutions, though less so today. What is being called into question today, however, is the nature of this contract; in other words whether it is freely entered into, open to negotiation, or can be withdrawn from. The notion of a fair exchange is also being called into question – what exactly does the service-user get out of it? Ideas that the service provider can offer a good deal in exchange for users surrendering their rights is certainly something that we would not accept readily, given some of the accounts we have of life in institutions.

The notion of a 'social contract' in which people get together for mutual benefit is perhaps being replaced with another version, the simple commercial contract. Here, a number of moves have been made to recast the relationship between service-user and provider as one in which market place rules apply. The service-user or consumer looks at whether the service offered for sale is worth buying, in much the same way as a car or a washing machine is viewed in a saleroom. If it looks appropriate, then the consumer goes ahead and buys it.

The idea of consumerism is evident in a number of government reports and policy statements. In the UK examples include, the NHS and Community Care Act of 1990, in which explicit reference was made to consumer power and ideas of choice and control. Le Grand (1990), however, has referred to this as a 'quasi-market', in the sense that the mechanisms which are assumed to govern and regulate the business market are not in place. The service-users as consumers, for example, are not always purchasing care directly unless they have sufficient resources. In other situations care is purchased on their behalf by a range of different agencies, for example health sector trusts, purchasing groups, social services departments and, even in the private sector, insurance companies. This proxy purchasing clearly contains the possibility of disempowerment of individuals as these agencies develop block contracts, set standards and constraints, or develop criteria for access and allocation, which may not coincide with the wishes of the individual.

Furthermore, the free-market notion of consumerism rests on the idea that the consumers have a clear set of preferences and views and, indeed, know what they want. Again, in the care market, this is by no means certain – service-users may not necessarily know what the options are or have criteria by which to compare them. Development of informed choice for service-users may require more than the handing out of glossy brochures, as in a car showroom, because of the complexities of what is available and what is needed. As individuals differ in circumstances and goals, then these differences are likely to be played out as a process of tailoring, adaptation and negotiation, rather than straightforward choosing.

This all suggests that using services is different from, say, buying a car. Cars are well understood items which we are likely to have some ideas about and which come with information. Care is not always understood; we may come to it suddenly or without thinking about it, and information may be hard to find or understand. Perhaps most importantly, buying a car is about acquiring a material object to carry out specified functions; purchasing care is more about embarking on a series of relationships which can profoundly shape the ways in which we carry out all activities of living and how we view ourselves and others. It is potentially much more important and complex than buying a car. The extreme criticism of consumerism in general, of course, is that it is naïve to assume that any consumer of anything has access to valid and reliable information that has not been filtered through the hands of some interested party.

These caveats about consumerism in care, however, do not really undermine the notion of empowerment – consumerism just seems like a particularly awkward way of addressing imbalances of power; one that is likely to create a whole set of different problems. These are not just pragmatic problems about, say, educating and training service-users to ask the right questions and make sound choices, but they are also philosophical problems about how we view the process of providing and using care services. Placing it in the stark language of commercial transactions certainly flags up the ideal of the service-user as being empowered to make decisions about care, to accept or refuse care, or to request particular forms of care. What it does not do, however, is address issues of power at an interpersonal level, or indeed acknowledge the interactional relationship aspect of care in any detail. As discussed in Chapter 6, the interpersonal dimensions of power have a strength beyond that of organisational structure and mechanisms for regulation.

There are, however, other discussions about empowerment which do not resort to the consumer model and which are based more on seeing care as a partnership between service-users and service providers. These arguments stay closer to the idea of a social contract, where exchange is based on identification of mutual benefits. This type of contract carries with it the obligation for all parties to make clear what these benefits, and costs, might be – they are not, apparently, as obvious as in the commercial contract. The process of making benefits obvious, however, often seems to be a bit one-sided – the benefits to the service-user are laid out, but those for the service provider are less clear. At one level, the benefits to the service provider might be given a gloss in terms of job satisfaction. This would sound something like, 'If you fulfil your part of the partnership then you will improve your quality of life and I will find my job more rewarding.' This move is interesting in that it implies that the service provider is entirely motivated by a desire to meet the needs of others; to see them get better, return home or whatever. As such, it claims a moral status for the service provider which may well repay further examination. A more subtle statement is one that goes, 'If you fulfil your role in this partnership, then the service will run smoother and will be able to help more people.' This statement again assumes that the function of the service is to help people, but is also using a form of utilitarian argument to suggest that the actions of the service-user might not be for the greater good. This type of statement not only claims the high moral ground for the service and service provider, but it also indicates ways in which the service-users might be construed as occupying the low moral ground – selfishly insisting on their preferences to the detriment of others. A related, and perhaps more honest, argument is to say, 'If you comply with this contract, then my job will be easier.' This at least recognises the possibility that service providers might be motivated by the desire to get through the day in a relatively stress-free way.

These variations on the social contract represent different types of corruption of the idea of empowerment. There are different pressures being brought to bear on the service-user which serve only to reinforce the fundamental paradox of any form of empowerment which is in the gift of service providers. If the terms of this empowerment are set by the provider, empowerment is compromised. At an even more fundamental level, if the decision to empower or not is in the hands of the service provider, then there is a contradiction in the process, especially if what power is given can also be taken away.

Perhaps the greatest corruption of the idea of empowerment lies in the strategy which effectively turns the tables entirely on the service-user, a move which can happen without any of the players anticipating it. It happens when an undercurrent of the empowerment goals is the idea that power brings responsibility. When power is handed over to service-users, therefore, sneaked in with this Trojan horse is the accompanying idea that a set of responsibilities is handed over too. Not only are the service-users free to make decisions, but they must take the blame if things go wrong. If the process is malevolently managed, the service provider can construct a situation where the power to actually make a success of things is restricted and failure is almost inevitable – a perverse interpretation of the social contract. An example would be to say to someone, 'You can provide your own care, but we won't give you any resources or advice.' When everything goes wrong, it is then easy to argue that these persons could not take responsibility for themselves and could not use the power that had been given to them wisely or well. From there it is easy to argue that they would be better off if someone else took over and made decisions for them.

Notions of empowerment are often mixed up with this parental view. The tensions between the rhetoric of empowerment for service-users, and the firmly entrenched idea that they are not really capable enough to deal with the responsibility, emerge in many different guises and under many different headings. Interestingly, both imperatives can be seen as essentially benevolent – it is not necessarily the case that parentalism is adopted through the worst of motives; sometimes it is a genuinely caring and concerned response to perceived difficulties.

To explore this puzzle further, examining the debates around risk and safety is an instructive exercise. These debates involve some consideration of ideas and concepts of freedoms and rights, yet this is often forgotten in the rush to estimate risk and develop strategies for risk management. It is as if the response of the organisation is decided before the basic principles which should inform action are debated. An overview of what could be discussed about freedom and risk is presented next.


## FREEDOM AND RISK

An important conceptual distinction to make in any debate is the difference between positive and negative freedoms. In other words, freedoms can be positive in that they are freedoms to do something: go for a walk, eat breakfast at midnight, vote, or access health care. Negative freedoms are freedoms to not have things inflicted upon oneself: freedom from injustice, coercion, discomfort, or injury. Many discussions about freedoms tend to concentrate on negative freedoms, establishing what people ought to be free from. This may be because it is easier to get some sort of consensus about negative freedoms and it is easier to make a case for them based on notions of the basic conditions necessary for an acceptable life.

Where things become more complicated, however, is where we start to think about positive freedoms. These have a profound political resonance and entire political movements have been galvanised by ideas of positive freedoms: to vote, to have a decent wage, or to have educational opportunities, for example. There is a corresponding political and ethical movement against such positive freedoms, however, which seems to be based on ideas of self-help and self-sufficiency, or can be formulated as some sort of meritocratic position. In essence this is: as long as negative freedoms are established, i.e. no-one unduly interferes with you, the rest is down to your own efforts and talents. To establish positive freedoms universally would undermine this idea of merit being the basis for their enjoyment.

The complexities of freedoms, then, are subtle, and in these debates there are many echoes of the debates that we have had elsewhere in this book, about models of practice and management, for example. What we need to do here, however, is connect them up to some everyday dilemmas that service providers are likely to face. Focusing round the issue of risk is one way to do this – as practice seems more and more mindful of risk issues, risk assessment and risk management being terms in frequent use, it is probably timely for this to be a starting point for an exploration of freedoms in institutional care.

There are many definitions and ideas about risk, but one of the most common approaches is summed up by The Royal Society (1992), as follows:

> ... risk as the probability that a particular adverse event occurs during a stated period of time, or results from a particular challenge. As a probability in the sense of statistical theory risk obeys all the formal laws of combining probabilities.

This statement about risk sets it in a rational and even mathematical framework. Risks of adverse events can be calculated if enough information is known about the variables involved. A number of authors have elaborated on and challenged this model, observing that it takes an awful lot for granted. It assumes a causality in human events which many would argue is spurious – life is much more random and chaotic than this. Another comment is that the degree of harm that any adverse event can cause is very much open to individuals' subjective feelings and is, therefore, impossible to calculate across groups, which is how mathematical risk frameworks are often used. Yet another critique comes from those who argue that the model is unilinear in that it only deals with one risk and set of probabilities at a time, whereas in real life risks are multiple and played off against each other. An example would be someone recovering from an operation, who has to balance the risk of exercising causing pain and making their sutures inflamed, and the risks of inactivity leading to a range of complications such as joint stiffness and chest infections. The particular balance of physical factors is also complicated by a range of social factors – the person may have a particular set of social circumstances, such as pressures from work or family responsibilities, that make one set of events more adverse than another, and in addition there are individual differences in attitudes to health, coping mechanisms and self-image. For an overview of these debates see Heyman (1998).

Despite these criticisms, the mathematical model of risk is a popular one with service managers, particularly those concerned with trying to prevent harm coming to service-users. This concern may be a genuine, if parental, worry that clients should be safe and well while they use the service and that the service should be able to identify potential risks to clients and safeguard against them. A more cynical concern might be about the possible consequences if an organisation were to be portrayed as failing in its duty of care. If a risk assessment has been carried out, and the organisational procedures followed in light of the assessment results, then it is possible to disclaim any culpability if a client then comes to harm.

The problem is, with both of these approaches, that if risk assessment is over-cautious, or if the organisational response is over-protective, then the freedom of clients can be compromised. While some may see the problem from the other side, where risk assessment and management are lax and clients are, therefore, not safeguarded, it is arguable that too vigorous a risk assessment may well have just as serious consequences. Given that the response to risk is largely to do with restricting activity in order to reduce probability of adverse events, such restrictions can represent significant losses of freedom.

Here, the idea of positive and negative freedoms provides an interesting approach to thinking about this. Curtailment of activity can be seen as an infringement of negative freedoms, in that people should not be restricted or subject to the orders of others. It can also be seen as an infringement of positive freedoms in that people should have the freedom to participate in activities that they want to participate in, and should have the freedom to make decisions about their activity and act on them. This freedom to make decisions is perhaps the key issue here, for of course the very fact that someone else has carried out a risk assessment on someone's behalf indicates that there is a view that the person's ability to do this for himself or herself is in question. The legitimacy and validity of this view is, of course, a matter for debate and previous sections of this book have explored this from a number of different angles. In this chapter, the idea comes up under parentalism, and in the chapter on models of practice (Chapter 5) it comes up under discussions of practice as benevolence. What we have is an argument which seems more like a tautology. It goes something like this: 'These persons are in an institution because they are unable to resolve their problems. The evidence for their inability to resolve their problems is the fact that they are in an institution.'

This parentalism, of course, focuses on one set of risks to the neglect of noticing another set of consequences. The risks that the institution or its agents might identify may be about short-term or immediate harms – clients may have accidents, be unable to care for themselves or whatever, and there is a probability that direct physical or psychological harm may ensue. There are a set of other harms, however, which are sometimes described as iatrogenic, in other words problems induced by the method of treating problems. Thus, if someone is unable to manage the household and spends time in some form of institutional care because of this, the experience may well make him or her even less likely to manage the household in the future. The experience of institutional care can be de-skilling and disempowering in many ways and creates a whole new set of risks and problems.

Notions of freedom, then, are compromised by notions of risk, especially where risk becomes the guide for institutional practice. Freedom as a guide for practice moves us on from this defensive position, but it then becomes important to address both negative and positive freedoms. Ultimately, however, these debates about risk and freedom can only be set out as broad principles and must have their start and endpoints with the service-user. We have argued that notions of risk are unique and individual, and that people weigh and balance competing risks and judge their impact in different ways. This makes it important that if someone starts to assess risks on behalf of anyone else, then this process must involve the service-users, if only in the way that an effort is made to see situations from their perspective.

The rhetoric of client-centred risk assessment and, indeed, the ideas about freedoms that it links to can be challenged by observations that at least some clients seem incapable of having these sorts of debate. Sometimes this challenge can be examined and found wanting, because it rests on assumptions made about the abilities of clients which have little evidence to support them. In some cases, however, there are obvious and genuine problems in handing over decisions to clients, because their health or functioning is in such a state as to make it very difficult to establish their preferences or feel sure that they have been able to understand their dilemma. Even where cognitive competence is not in question, it may be the case that issues are so complex and require such a degree of specialist knowledge that it is difficult for anyone to make a decision – say, for example about legal or medical questions.

This does not necessarily mean that freedom and self-determination should be taken away entirely and immediately – autonomy is not necessarily a property that we have or do not have. It is not the case that we either do everything for ourselves in absolute freedom, or that we do nothing without the control of others. Collopy (1988), for example, in his discussion about autonomy in older people, argues that there are a number of freedoms, including the freedom to delegate decision-making to others. The crucial point is that this delegation is directed by the service-users and is not a process imposed on them or instigated without any negotiation at all. The grey area between absolute freedom and absolute lack of freedom is the area that most of us live in most of the time, and it is a mistake to think that service-users are not in there with us. The problem that we have, though, is working out these shades of grey and what we should do at different points and in different positions.

A central issue, and one that we have only touched on so far, is about what we think we are negotiating with, that is the nature of the service-users. This is not something as simple as whether they are ill or not, or what sort of problems they have, or what type of personality they display, but a much more fundamental question about their status as a person. So far in this book, we have talked about service-users as being 'discredited', sometimes because of their service use. What we mean by this is that service-users can be seen as less than persons because of their supposed problems or situations: these can be construed as deficits which reduce their claims to be autonomous rational agents. This permits or justifies service providers in acting for service-users, either benignly or corruptly, because they are somehow not fully developed humans. We have heard service-users described as being 'like children' or, in very punitive regimes, as being 'like animals', and both of these descriptions emphasise their lack of adult status. Seeing clients as not-persons, then, allows a whole raft of practices to take place – Evers' (1981) description of the care of older people as 'warehousing' vividly illustrates this process. Notions of personhood, then, have important consequences for the way in which care is shaped, and an exploration of the philosophical debates about personhood can be instructive.

## PERSONHOOD

One way to differentiate or categorise philosophical theories of personhood is to put them under two headings: 'normative' and 'non-normative' (Reed and Ground, 1997). While these categories may be more about the emphasis of different theories rather than absolute differences, nevertheless they are still useful. Normative theories, as the title indicates, suggest that to be a person an entity needs to comply with norms of personhood, in other words be broadly in line with other things that we call persons. This can involve characteristics such as language use, rationality, or autonomy. One of the problems with these theories is that, depending on the picture of the norm, exclusions can seem very difficult to justify. Language use, for example, is a normal characteristic of things we call people, but the inability to use language does not seem sufficient grounds to see a human being as a non-person. Another problem is that they see these characteristics as being intrinsic properties of the human being that exhibits them, rather than properties that are, in part, socially constructed. Autonomy, for example, is not a property or characteristic of a person, like their height or weight, but is something which is negotiated with others.

Non-normative theories involve consideration of the conditions of personhood, and a particular strand of enquiry involves looking at the impact of changes over time on the status of personhood. In other words, these theories are concerned with finding out what can change without personhood being affected and what must remain stable. In this line of investigation there are a number of 'mind-experiment' or hypothetical situations that are presented. For example, it might be asked whether, if a person's entire body is destroyed and then replicated, say through a machine something like those in science fiction programmes where people are 'beamed up' to various places, then would we still consider them to be the same person? There are other more prosaic examples – does someone with total amnesia, who has no sense of identity, no memories and no personal history to reflect on, still count as a person, particularly if we hold to the idea that what makes a person is precisely these memories and experiences?

These questions translate into care situations. Is someone still the same person if they respond entirely differently to the world, and in ways which are directly contradictory to previous responses? For some people with mental health problems, this may seem to be the case and if we feel that they are not the same person, then we might ask whether they are now a different person, or even a person at all. If we apply normative theories we might look at behaviour, say language use, and think that because the service-user does not display normal characteristics of a person, then they are not one.

Determining what is a person is one debate, but resolving this is only part of the personhood question. We then need to ask how we treat humans who are persons and humans who are not. If, for example, we decide that a human in a persistent vegetative state does not meet our definition of a person, for whatever reason, then we still need to decide how we should treat this entity and what respect or care is due or not due to it. We do not make an automatic move from deciding that someone is not a person to deciding that we owe them no duty of care. Debates on euthanasia demonstrate this quite clearly. Where someone is diagnosed as being in a persistent vegetative state, this does not automatically mean that withdrawing treatment or active ending of life is condoned. That we still have a lengthy debate indicates something about the way that personhood extends beyond the individual and is something that is the product of social relationships. The responsibilities and obligations of these relationships, therefore, are not automatically cancelled or negated by changes in the entity we see as a person.

Personhood, then, is not an all or nothing state; there are different degrees and forms. While we have problems in thinking about personhood as being 'switched on' at some point in our development, it is even more difficult to think of it as being switched off at some point. This suggests that ideas of personhood, particularly normative ideas, should not be a driving force behind care, and that we need to think more broadly about how we interact as human beings rather than be eager, in a range of informal and covert ways as well as in more official mechanisms, to detect 'non-personhood' in service-users, and respond with parentalism and abuses of freedom.

## Conclusions

This chapter has outlined very briefly a range of ethical and moral debates which seem to us to be particularly relevant to issues in institutional care. We have engaged to some extent in using these philosophical concepts and frameworks as tools to examine care and to draw together some of the ideas and issues that we have raised elsewhere in this book. The final chapter moves on to a consideration of how these concepts might be brought to bear on institutional care in more formal ways, through the development of strategies such as ethical audits.

# 8 Ethical audit: a way forward

| |
|---|
| Audit methodology |
| Basis for a model of ethical audit |
| Summary |

A number of themes have recurred throughout this book; ideas about the dynamics of work and care in institutional settings. The premise that we began with was that care in institutions will always form part of the range of services offered to clients. To argue that they are places of deprivation and neglect, and that they should be closed down, simply does not help. There are concerns about what would replace them – community care is by no means unproblematic, as we have discussed in Chapters 1 and 2, and cannot be treated as a panacea for all the problems reported in institutional care. This means that we have to engage with these problems in a more proactive and reflective way and also to see the potentials of institutions or, perhaps more accurately, re-discover them.

In Chapters 3 and 4 we explored specific issues and theories in relation to practice, and in Chapters 5, 6, and 7 we discussed generalities in the context of developing meta-understandings of care practice. We have seen from the material on theories of management that embedded systems can be of fundamental importance in ensuring what the baseline standards are, and significant in achieving consistency in their application. This is not to stifle creativity, for it is part of the process to make certain that it flourishes. However, it is to prevent the necessity for creating new systems from the start every time and by implication, therefore, freeing up energies for the demanding tasks of the moment. Quite apart from any issue of standards for internal purposes, service-users are entitled to be enabled to know what standards of functioning are applied. Applying the principles of consumerism to care services is no longer an optional activity; it is now a requirement. What we wish to explore now are ways of deriving some notions of practice usefulness from this material. In particular, we have argued that it is important to develop systems which can redress centrally emerging themes of power imbalance, especially in terms of the contract between service provider and service-user.

Therefore, outlining a possible framework for action is the work of this chapter. It is useful to think of the processes of opening up care at two levels:

the institutional, or organisational, level and the practice, or individual level. We are concerned with institutional care and the elements of institutional care that make it different from care carried out in other settings or contexts. However, we need to move away from the idea that good care is simply a matter of individual and personal behaviour. It is undoubtedly true that the personal attributes that practitioners bring to care are vitally important, but to lose a sense of practice context is ultimately unproductive. Practitioners can be exhorted to be better people, but if the organisation does not become a better organisation, it is difficult to see how this will create anything other than frustration in staff.

Nevertheless, in thinking about how best to achieve change we should exercise caution, since many of the good-practice mantras such as dignity, respect and self-determination have often been promoted within a working culture which does not necessarily apply them internally. And, as we are reminded by Nocon and Qureshi (1996), agencies can regard service-users as social or physical casualties rather than citizen-consumers. Within the developing political context of social exclusion, it may be a moot point as to whether or not, for example, the proliferation within health and social care systems of 'customer care' services act in the interests of the provider by filtering access, or whether they serve an inclusive function by facilitating access for the service-user. Examples of the ambiguity of professional response to the Patients' Charter are explored by Anandale in Allott and Robb (1998). More specifically for our purposes, the presentation of 'front of house' reception in many residential care homes may, or may not, reflect the overall environment beyond the entrance hall.

One potential way forward lies in the adoption of the mechanisms of ethical audit. In the following section, we review the contribution which audit methodology can make in creating links between the person, the provider and the provision in a meaningful way that is sustainable both in ideological and practice terms. We shall then progress to considering a values-driven, ethical approach to audit.

## Audit methodology

We have already referred elsewhere to a range of instruments which have been developed to assure care standards, and have acknowledged the significance of their contribution. We propose that another system which can make a positive contribution to standards of care is to apply the process of audit methodology. This is not yet another tool, or technology, to be reified for its own sake, but instead can be used as a concrete method for establishing the principles of good practice within the institution. It also provides a vehicle to aid the reflective practitioner in operating within a framework of negotiated consent. In this sense it may more effectively perform the function which has been projected on to other approaches which have subsequently been seen as more tokenistic within the care sector (for example the externally imposed policing approach to ensuring minimum standards). If that is its purpose, what do we mean by audit methodology? In this section we explore some of the definitions and usages.

The traditional model of audit is essentially an examination of records, though we do not use the term in quite such a limited way. Apart from the obvious general applications to finance and contract compliance, the term is also used with quite specific applications in health care: medical audit, clinical audit, nursing audit. Nor, for our present purposes, are we concerned with a narrowly biomedical approach. It is also pertinent to note that these other professional usages can by no means be seen in a simplistic way. For example, in the arena of accountancy, as a process for exploring the financial state of health of an organisation, the term 'audit' must be qualified. An examination of the annual accounts may be described variously as a traditional audit, an independent examination, or a regulated audit. Each one of these approaches has particular methodologies, strengths and purposes. And so it is when reviewing the functional health of an institution: the variety of instruments each have differing strengths and purposes. Whilst an audit may often be used to describe a retrospective function, we are concerned with interactive, ongoing applications, i.e. a systematic, quality-of-life assessment and one which might also usefully incorporate a diagnostic function.

The work of the Audit Commission is well known and respected and its activities are much more diverse than merely a narrow value-for-money accountancy exercise. However, in concerning itself with both practice issues and public expenditure interests, there will always be questions concerning priorities and motivation. How far, for example, the Griffiths Report (1988) was driven by structural, financial or practice imperatives will always remain open to debate, notwithstanding the specificity of its terms of reference. In tracing the developments from that report through to the White Paper *Caring for People* (Department of Health, 1989) and on to the 1990 NHS and Community Care Act with its split timescale of implementation, myriad factors contributed to the eventual and continuing impact on practice. It should be recognised that there exist similar tensions within an institutional setting. One way of minimising such 'fogging' might, through negotiation, be to articulate clearly the various functions of the processes in the context of the general stakeholders' contributions.

Audit can also be associated with the development of a range of assessment approaches, from the specific function of clinical monitoring (for example in health), to the needs-led assessments of community care, the notion of audit-trail as a vehicle for demonstrating quality assurance, and the overall functions of meta-monitoring QA systems. Nocon and Qureshi (1996, pp. 144–5) usefully define audit as 'a cycle of activity which involves the systematic review of practice, development of possible improvements, implementation of these, and further review'. It is worth expanding these essential characteristics a little. The key descriptor is arguably the 'cycle'. There is little practice value to be had from merely developing a descriptive, retrospective inventory. Therefore any audit must:

- within the contexts of good-practice values and especially of stakeholder participation, ensure that it does not become a linear device which fails to return to the point at which it started;
- be rigorous and exhaustive in its processes, which should be developed in consultation with the stakeholders;
- be clear that its primary purpose is to contribute to the maintenance of good practice and develop proposals for making and implementing improvements;
- be open and explicit concerning its process for managing outcomes (there is little point in producing a detailed report of data and analysis if there is no mechanism for addressing findings);
- have a loop-back mechanism which not only keeps the whole process under systematic review but particularly focuses on the progress of implementing change.

These are demanding requirements and possibly need to be set in the context of more specific perspectives. Wilson (1997, p. 272) presents a model of 'variance analysis', which looks at identifying where and why events do not occur within the agreed 'pathway'. This approach provides a simple form of record keeping which may be custom designed and which can be used to provide the data that establish whether or not agreed practice is maintained. Øvretveit *et al.* (1997, pp. 12 and 98) explore a networking framework for auditing patient or client involvement. The major orientation of this model is towards looking at patient/client involvement in their service. However, in promoting the significance of consultation, the questions which are suggested are identified and asked by the staff team, rather than in collaboration with the service-user. Whilst it is important to understand the professionals' contribution to the service, this staff-driven approach seems to neglect the establishment of the service-users' role in contributing to the development of the audit mechanism. Reigate (in Davies, 1997, p. 218) also talks about a model of networking (micro, mezzo, macro) analysis, but is conscious of the workers' duty to be aware of client perceptions and how networks can both obstruct or enable coping. In this respect the three-stage model does give some indication of how to locate the various constituent parts. The micro level allows us to focus on the individual's (for example, in our instance the service-user's) personal network. The mezzo level forms a link between the individual and their wider, external needs (for example, in terms of external support). The macro level is more concerned with relationships with more formal external activities. Whilst this model is derived from a social networking perspective, it can be usefully modified to provide a multi-level structure for exploring issues.

Raynor (also in Davies, 1997, pp. 306–9) deals with the introduction and development of national standards in the probation service, posing some interesting questions about how far the functions of national standards lead to the sort of practice with which we are concerned. Although this debate might at first sight appear distant from our consideration of institutional care, there are common themes. In the first instance, the probation service has experienced the ambiguous dualism of whether or not it is a criminal justice agency, or social welfare agency, or both. This is not a new phenomenon in spite of its restructuring and re-orientation, both of which arguably owe more to political frameworks of reference than to a concern with good practice. The functions of institutional care are similarly ambiguous, partly from the health care/social care dimensions, but also in respect of precise definitions of purpose. Secondly, there is the vexed question of whether or not regulatory and audit systems which are designed to ensure standards actually do contribute towards the development and maintenance of good practice, or whether they might, of themselves, create a style of approach which is antithetical to such goals. This dilemma reminds us that any system should have an integral mechanism to guard against any such possibility.

In Raynor's terms, in striving for a predictable and accountable level of service, we must not strangulate the very qualities of which we are in search. Equally however, we must respond positively to the negativities which proclaim that nothing can, or ever will, work.

## CREATION OF AN ETHOS

In many respects the adoption of a particular system for ensuring acceptable levels of quality of life in social and health care, whilst not an arbitrary choice, is a matter for which there cannot be prescribed answers. Rather like other aspects of consumerism, there are a range of issues to be taken into account and choices will be made on the basis of a number of locally determined perspectives (for example size of institution, levels of dependency, budget). However, there does need to be an acknowledgement that the adoption of a system, whichever it might be, is necessary. The consumer is so often in a vulnerable and less powerful situation that to leave it to them or their carers to satisfy themselves as to standards is simply not an acceptable option. We are too familiar with many of the dynamics of dependency to take such risks.

It is also equally mistaken to imagine the reverse to be acceptable, i.e. that the institution can take on all the responsibilities associated with the maintenance of quality standards. Whilst we have elsewhere argued that standards are too important to be left to imposition from external regulators, such regulators are a hugely important link in the overall process. In an operational environment where there are no internalised controls, they may be the only part of that process. If an ethos of principled self-monitoring and control is one effective way to ensure that good standards exist, that ethos must underpin effective structures. In turn, those structures must be both inward and outward looking. We have in our opening and subsequent chapters demonstrated that the perverse manifestations of institutional living emerge in an environment where there is neglect from the outside world and power is unevenly distributed internally. By ethical audit we mean the adoption of both a philosophy and processes which will enable all stakeholders in the life of the institution to contribute to the setting and maintenance of acceptable standards. If we return to Wilmot's (1997) use of the word 'stakeholder', then we also endow the consumer with a certain enhanced set of rights and responsibilities in this respect. The process must therefore be inclusive.

We have also established that we believe that the process must be both interactive and responsive. The final question here is to think about to which levels and standards aspirations should be matched. Often in the language of quality assurance, the words 'acceptable minimum standards' arise, and this presents a particular problem of definition. Minimum standards are defined and desired in different ways by different sectors and their constituents. If the corollary is that there is also to be found an inventory headed 'acceptable maximum standards', then no such document exists. It is always possible to challenge assumptions on which standards are based, but ultimately any firm decision should be substantially informed and owned by the particular stakeholders. The populist paraphrase of Bowlby's (1953) original view, that the worst natural parent must be better than the best substitute home, is no longer a sustainable view, and in terms of our awareness of knowledge of elder abuse (e.g. Biggs et al., 1995) neither is it applicable in broader terms to the care of older people. Paradoxically, the standards of care debate is not one which is clear even in terms of family care, or self-care in independent living. The principal reason for this is that lifestyle and standards are dependent upon multiple variables, not least of which is a consideration of risk factors, as we have discussed in Chapter 7. Therefore, any fixing of standards in a particular case must take into account dependency, independency and interdependency issues.

## SPECIFIC APPROACHES TO AUDIT

There is an increasing realisation of the importance of the ethical components of audit. In arenas as diverse as business and accountancy, it is acknowledged that it is no longer satisfactory to ignore the ethical dimension and there is a growing literature which develops these themes. Looking closer to home, in the field of health education, Duncan (1995) has drawn attention to an increasing awareness of moral problems in a paper entitled 'Ethical audit: should it concern health promoters?', though some of the conclusions drawn, for example that solutions will not always be found, may appear unsatisfactory in our quest for better practice. Nevertheless, this does at least point to an understanding that there are problems which need to be addressed. However, there do not appear to be any fully developed models of ethical audit designed for the purposes of exploring institutional care practice. Therefore we have to turn to material which is as closely analogous as possible, and a useful starting point is to consider clinical audit in health care. One definition of clinical audit, derived from the NHS Executive (Mann, 1996), reads thus:

> a clinically led initiative which seeks to improve the quality and outcome of patient care through structured peer review whereby clinicians examine their practices and results against agreed standards and modify their practice where indicated.

This is a helpful place to start for a number of reasons. Firstly, it should be noted that this is a generic definition, both in terms of reference and application, and one which embraces a quite specific focus. Earlier definitions tended to vary according to who might be involved in the process. For example, a report by the National Council for Hospice and Specialist Palliative Care Services (Higginson, 1992) carried five separate definitions: medical audit, clinical audit, nursing audit, prospective audit, and retrospective audit. It is not necessary to repeat here all five of their different definitions, except to acknowledge that for the first category, medical audit, the report used the earlier 1989 definition of the Department of Health:

> The systematic critical analysis of the quality of medical care including the procedures used for diagnosis and treatment, the use of resources, and the resulting outcome and quality of life of the patient.
>
> (Department of Health, 1989)

There was a qualitatively different definition for nursing audit:

> The methods by which nurses compare their actual practice against pre-agreed guidelines and identify areas for improving their care.
>
> (Higginson, 1992, p. 5)

We would argue that the latter is more explicit and focused than the former, and that whilst this is by no means an easy task in any circumstances, the former moves into territory which is notoriously difficult to define. In particular, the medical definition covers a very broad spread of activities, some of which, such as 'quality of life', may not be capable of being satisfactorily determined. This is redolent of many of the health and social care reports which we have explored: generalised solutions to generalised problems rarely lead to satisfactory outcomes. Whilst we would not want to minimise the difficulties in implementing the nursing model, it at least possesses the merit of being capable of defining relatively tighter boundaries around relatively fewer potential variables. Therefore, it comes as no surprise that the more recent definition from the NHS Executive, cited previously, follows this pathway.

The impetus for nursing audit developed in the USA and derived from the quality assurance movement. It is pertinent to note that one of the seminal texts referred to following the NCHSPCS definition cited above was entitled *The Nursing Audit: Self-Regulation in Nursing Practice* (Phaneuf, 1976). It is worth quoting the opening remarks of this text:

> There is a social contract between society and the professions. Under its terms, society grants the professions authority over functions vital to itself and permits them considerable autonomy in the conduct of their own affairs. In return, the professions are expected to act responsibly, always mindful of the public trust. Self-regulation to assure quality in this performance is at the heart of this relationship. It is the authentic hallmark of a mature profession.                    (Phaneuf, 1976, p. xiii)

These words are as central to our own approach as when Donabedian wrote them more than 25 years ago as the foreword to Phaneuf's first edition. There is little merit in our recitation of the incantations of quality, professional responsibilities and self-regulation if we fail to develop mechanisms which are designed to test our performances in these, and other, respects. However, whilst it is both reassuring and constructive to return to this earlier work for an overview and to remind us of the ethics basis of the development, it is nonetheless necessary to acknowledge that Phaneuf's model was essentially a clinical audit which relied on a particularly circumscribed set of parameters and instruments. It did not set out actively to embrace general environmental or consumer perspectives, both of which are central to our concerns.

## IMPLEMENTING AUDIT

Returning to current views on clinical audit, it is very clear from the NHS Executive definition cited above that the focus on clinical audit as a means of self-regulation has become well established. However, it is also appropriate to define it by what it is not: it is neither intended to be an organisational or management audit, nor to serve the purposes of an externally imposed or managed audit. The notion of 'audit trail' may be a useful one, but again it is not the purpose of clinical audit to turn the exercise into a mere paper chase, no matter how valid a place such an activity might have in quality assurance terms. The literature of audit in general, and clinical audit in particular, all points to a process which, whilst it may be expressed in a variety of different ways, is usually described as cyclical, or circular, and tends to embrace the following components:

**Topics → Agreed criteria → Observation/Data collection → Comparison/reflection on practice against agreed criteria → Identification and agreement of necessary change → Implementation of change → Monitoring and re-audit → (Repeat cycle)**

Each of the above stages has attached to it an associated implementation methodology, usually together with a training or familiarisation and support process. However, useful as this model might be in the clinical health setting, a number of difficulties emerge in applying it to the health and social care context. This is partly because clinical audit in health occurs in multiple ways in relation to clinical specialisms, whose protocols have usually – though not always – become firmly established over time. They, therefore, deal with micro-aspects of the clinical context. It is also partly because the health setting, in its development of the clinical audit, has largely not addressed the matter of social, as opposed to clinical, perspectives.

An example of such an audit which reaches, or perhaps fails to reach, to the heart of institutional care, is the research report commissioned by SELHCA (Bennett *et al.*, 1995). Essentially, this study is concerned with an audit of the appropriateness of nursing home placements, and examined 157 clients who were admitted to 25 nursing homes from home, hospital or residential care, from a random sample from three London boroughs around 1993. It may not have been the commissioners' intention to obtain service-user perspectives, but this is an example of a study which fails to offer a vehicle for the voice of the resident. Whilst much of the study was concerned with conducting an audit trail of documentation, the researchers also 'assessed' 13 of the homes using the following headings (pp. 8–9):

- Personal autonomy
- Promotion of continence
- Optimising drug use
- Managing falls
- Pressure sores
- Environment and equipment
- Aids and adaptations
- Medical role.

Regrettably the report does not offer any substantive detail of the methodology used, but the results as reported are very limited and give a very clear picture of generalisation, with a predominant focus on the clinical aspects of care. Even those headings, such as the first and sixth headings above, which might appear to offer coverage of environmental and lived experiences of the care setting, failed to probe the residents' world from their own perspectives. The study also reported on differences between the homes in terms of 'quality issues' (pp. 925–9); again, neither the context nor definition of quality is developed within the report, but the headings under which it reported were:

- Management
- Staffing
- Decor
- Atmosphere
- Smell
- Dress of patients
- Food
- GP cover
- When a resident is about to die
- Documentation and general organisation
- Equipment.

The failure to define quality, or to link it to any recognisable quality-oriented model, renders virtually meaningless the brief commentaries which are made under each heading. The absence of any user-centred perspective is starkly demonstrated under 'When a resident is about to die', where the commentary deals exclusively with staff world perspectives and does not use the opportunity to comment on matters such as other residents' experiences of loss or mourning for their co-residents. This matter of 'quality' within the homes is summed up by three lines in the report's conclusions:

> Generally we found a reasonably good standard of care within most of the homes, but there were exceptions and we recommend that stricter quality standards are implemented. (p. 34)

It is quite difficult to understand how such a generalisation can be determined from the evidence contained within the report. More fundamentally, however, this example emphasises both the inappropriateness of drawing such qualitative conclusions from the audit and highlights ways in which reports can present broad, overview recommendations, apparently without giving any accompanying consideration to their capacity to be implemented.

## AN AMERICAN APPROACH

In contrast with the above example, the work of Moos (1974, 1987) and Moos and Lemke (1994) provides us with a highly detailed and structured account of social climate in group residences for older adults. In particular, the 1994 text focuses on factors which contribute to the quality of life for older people within the residential environment, especially the physical and social aspects. In their introductory chapter, which offers an intriguing brief history of residential care programmes for older people in the United States, the authors distinguish between two types of research: that which defines types and characteristics of group living, and that which explores the relationship between group housing and resident characteristics and outcomes. It is with this second group that we are concerned. Moos and Lemke, with their research team, studied more than 300 residential settings throughout the United States, basing their work upon three overarching conceptual assumptions:

- the need for new ways to characterise salient aspects of residential programmes;
- that a common conceptual framework might be used advantageously to evaluate residential programmes;
- that more emphasis should be placed on the process of matching personal and programme factors, and on the connections between person–environment congruence and resident outcomes.

Building on Moos's earlier work, Moos and Lemke developed an instrument which they called the Multiphasic Environmental Assessment Procedure (MEAP) to assess the group residential setting. The five component parts of MEAP provide an insight into what were considered to be the significant aspects of the environment (resident and staff characteristics, physical features, policies and services, and social climate) and are:

- The Resident and Staff Information Form: for measuring aspects of the suprapersonal environment, i.e. the sociodemographic characteristics of residents and staff.
- The Physical and Architectural Checklist: direct observation of the physical environment.
- The Policy and Programme Information Form: the policies and services as reported by appropriate staff and administrators.
- The Sheltered Care Environment Scale: an assessment of residents' and staff perceptions of identified characteristics of the social environment.
- The Rating Scale: external observers' assessments of the characteristics of the setting and of the residents' and staff functioning.

The language of this American text can fall strangely upon European ears. However, its very strangeness can act as a vehicle to make us stop and think about its meaning. Far too often we can come across the familiar and disregard it as commonplace, without really paying it the attention which it might merit. The fact that it takes a substantial text, such as this one, to present and discuss the evaluation methodology says something about its level of detail and, by implication, about the arena in which it operates. And the fact that in itself it represents a development of more than 20 years' work gives some indication of the complexity and sophistication of both the model and the authors' conclusions.

We would argue that the MEAP model both supports and represents much of the case which we have been making for the provision of a usable methodology of audit, though with a number of important provisos. In the first instance, Moos and Lemke are reporting on a substantial national survey involving a programme which is externally administered, notwithstanding the fact that there is a significant focus on insider contributions. Second, the obverse of the first, the process is not internally administered. Therefore one of our key requirements of user-ownership is not met. Third, there is an implicit though unquantified, except to a certain extent in terms of research programme funding, resource implication for the administration of the complex assessment instruments. Finally, there is some limited reference in the text to differential findings between the United States and the United Kingdom. Notwithstanding these issues, the approach represents a substantive initiative in terms of measuring and making sense of the lived experience of the institutional environment.

## VALUE OF AN AUDIT-BASED APPROACH

In closing this review of the meaning and purpose of audit, we would return to the work of Wardhaugh and Wilding (in Allott and Robb, 1998), who argued that the application of principles of enquiry can, at least, be helpful in identifying situations in which care systems might be at risk of becoming compromised. We would also argue that, conversely, there is similarly a duty for service providers to ensure that care environments offer a positive service. Within this context, the notion of audit has a concrete contribution to make. By this we mean the idea of audit as an instrument for enabling the positive development of good practice standards over and above notions of good-enough or minimum-acceptable levels of provision. To be effective, audit must contain an ethically aware component and be located in a conceptual awareness which has the capacity to be both focused and explicit in its requirements.

## Basis for a model of ethical audit

In this section we want to take some of the themes which we believe to be fundamental to developing practice and use them as a basis for exploring potential mechanisms for taking care forward. There is the idea of reification, that the institution becomes a 'thing in itself', rather than something which is created and maintained by people. Examples of this are where we hear people talking about 'the hospital' or 'the care home' as agents, with goals and behaviours. When people make comments such as 'this hospital doesn't like complaints', there is a subtle move away from the idea of the hospital as a building in which people provide care (as in 'this hospital doesn't have a casualty department') to an idea of the hospital which almost gives it a persona. This process of reification is common in institutions; indeed some would say that it is an enduring feature of institutional life, and there are many examples of affectionate reification, for example in school songs where pupils sing to the school as if it were a person.

Whilst such processes may contribute towards a feeling of belonging to those who live and work in institutions, there are, of course, a number of less positive consequences. The reification of the institution can often hide the real agents involved in the way that it operates, and provides a diversionary tactic for those who want to avoid criticism. If it is possible to lay the blame on the organisation rather than the individuals in it, then it becomes more difficult to change things, or to call people to account. This process is a disempowering one, as those who live and work in institutions become overwhelmed by the idea of the institution as the object that causes things to happen – an institution is much more difficult to pin down than the individuals within it.

Throughout this book we have tried to explore ways in which institutional care can be opened up for scrutiny and examination and what sorts of criteria this might involve. Taking a look at the institution as a place in which a range of people meet and act, rather than as a being in its own right, is one step towards this. Once we have moved beyond reification, however, we still need some sort of framework for looking – we need to be clear about what we are looking for and why, and how we should interpret information that we get through this process. We shall, therefore, build on our review of audit to consider a specific example of an ethical audit and the methodological issues that it raises.

## INSTITUTIONAL MECHANISMS FOR SCRUTINY

We have, above, outlined the principles behind tools such as quality assurance measures and audit, and of the importance of ideology in thinking about our values base. Here, we take those principles further to look at how they can be combined with discussions on the ethics and values of institutional care to provide a framework for examining what goes on in institutions and how practices might be changed.

The 'ethical audit' is an approach which has much potential. Most organisations display mission statements and charters about the service that they provide and the standards that they want these services to meet. These are based, implicitly or explicitly, on sets of values and models of care. The rhetoric of the mission statement, however, cannot be treated as an accurate description of what happens in an institution, because the practices of the institution may not match at all with what is written – it may have been developed in ignorance of actual behaviour in the institution, or in a spirit of naïve idealism. The mission statement cannot even be taken as a reflection of shared goals and values in the institution: if it is written by one group of people without consultation with others then it may reflect a particular view of the institution which is not shared very widely.

Mission statements, and other documents like them, can only be treated as a statement of aspirations reflecting a section of the people living and working in the institution. This does not make them valueless, but they are perhaps of less weight than their authors might hope. An ethical audit, however, can use them as a starting point for inquiry, and as a template against which to match the institution. If the match is not a close one, this does not automatically mean that the problem lies entirely in the institution or in the mission statement, and an ethical audit may help us to see how they can both be brought into closer alignment.

There are two main parts of an ethical audit as Henry (1995) has described it. The first is an investigation of the values in an institution, and the second is an exploration of how those values are manifested in practice. Other functions of an ethical audit are dependent on the needs of the organisation, for example it may serve to test the potential for change, to check out responses to developments internally or externally, or simply to increase self-awareness across an organisation of the values which it practices.

Investigating the values of an organisation, what they are and the extent to which they are shared, is the first stage of an ethical audit and it is an extremely difficult one. There are problems in engaging in any information gathering which does not ensure anonymity, or where respondents may feel uncomfortable about revealing their views to a researcher. Questionnaire-style methods do not necessarily solve the problems either. As Campbell (1995) has noted, the development of a questionnaire needs to take into account issues of language and presentation. Constructing questions which are not loaded towards a particular response is very difficult but, if this is not done, the questionnaire might simply be asking people if they support the ethical equivalent of motherhood and apple pie and obtain correspondingly bland answers in response.

There are other issues about developing tools for this stage of an ethical audit that become even more pressing if a questionnaire-style approach is used. A questionnaire, or any other type of structured approach, needs a starting point and how this starting point is framed and presented impacts on responses. Asking people whether they agree or disagree with a statement seems a relatively unproblematic strategy, until you start to think through the composition of the statements and from where they have come. A statement such as 'this institution should provide individualised care' is not simply a neutral idea for people to comment on, but is a statement that has come from some overview of the institutional issues and the judgement of the audit team that this is a key issue. It is always possible that a different analysis would have come up with a different set of key issues, and so ethical audit must be clear in the way that it arrives at this point, where questions are formulated, and must be open itself to challenge.

In view of these issues, the Ethical and Values Audit (EVA) team at the University of Central Lancashire developed a range of strategies for their ethical audit of the University. In addition to a questionnaire, the team used an 'ethics hotline' for people to leave anonymous comments. From these, a range of case studies were developed. The team also used interviews and a form of ethical grid which resembled repertory grid methods. This 'values identification grid' explored the way that respondents categorised ethical concepts and values (Henry, 1995). Individuals were asked to give a positive or negative score to themselves and 17 other roles (for example a line manager or student). These scores were in relation to how the person or role was rated along a series of constructs, such as trustworthy/untrustworthy and open/closed. These constructs were derived from the questionnaires and interviews that had been carried out, and respondents were also invited to elicit their own. In addition, the EVA team examined university policy documents and statements to identify the ethical principles they contained. The variety of approaches that the EVA team used reflects the complexity of the ethical audit task – where values are private and personal, or where those who hold them may find it difficult to articulate them, then finding out about them is extremely difficult.

The next stage of ethical audit, where the playing out of values in practice is explored, is equally difficult. It involves a critique and modelling of the values uncovered in the first stage and then a process whereby these values are presented as activities or behaviours. For example, a set of values around open communication with clients could be translated into a set of activities such as holding meetings with clients, passing on information to them, making information available to them, or directing them towards sources of advice. Exploring how these values are translated into practice, therefore, would involve looking at practice to see how often these things happened, and also how they happened. It might not be enough simply to note the frequency of meetings; it might also be necessary to find out what their content was and how they were managed.

The methods used in ethical audit depend, therefore, on a combination of the aspects that need to be studied and the ethics of the audit itself; in other words, whether the methods are intrusive or damaging to participants. Research codes of ethics indicate that confidentiality should be maintained, for example, and this may have major implications for the way in which data are collected and presented. Another set of issues is about the scope and range of data collection. Given that every aspect of an institution or organisation has a bearing on, and relationship to, the values of that organisation, the potential scope is vast. For this reason, an ethical audit may focus in on a specific area, say, for example, equal opportunities, and focus mainly on recruitment policy and practice.

This focusing down may also reflect the process of commissioning or instigating an ethical audit. The decision to engage in this process is usually made by particular people in an organisation, and may be in response to a particular issue that they have identified. A number of consequences might result: the identified issue may not turn out to be as crucial as was first thought, or its importance might not be recognised beyond the groups of people directly involved in instigating the audit. Again, this suggests that a degree of flexibility in the audit is essential. Perhaps more problematically, the process of commissioning an audit may set off a range of organisational tremors which may have an impact on both the exercise and on the organisation.

If an audit is seen as a management plot to identify malcontents (and this may be particularly crucial if the organisation is awash with talk about redundancy or 'rationalisation') then a whole set of pressures is generated as respondents try to guess what the 'right' answers will be to any questions they are asked. Audits may be interpreted as punitive or coercive, or as an attempt to settle disputes, and these interpretations may not only have an effect on the audit, but also on the organisation as a whole. What might be conceived of as an exercise in openness may turn into an exercise that encourages defensiveness.

These, then, are some of the broad points about ethical audits. Accounts of their use in a range of different settings are available and, although the literature is not huge, it is growing. Applying the principles of ethical audit to care institutions, however, may present particular challenges. First, no audit would be complete without looking at the service-user's view, but this may encourage the idea of the audit as setting the staff and the client groups in opposition to each other, where the service-users 'inform' on the staff. Staff might feel very unhappy about the process if they see service-users as being unreliable or invalid in their views (see Chapter 7). Service-users may be reluctant to comment for a range of reasons: feelings of support for the staff, or anxiety about repercussions for themselves.

Second, if institutions are largely self-contained, in that they have little traffic with the outside world, the language and customs of the institution can become entrenched. This makes it difficult for audit teams to map out values, decide which are key, or to identify activities in which they might be demonstrated. Furthermore, such rigidity may make the development of changes in strategies as a result of the audit extremely difficult.

Third, an ethical audit can present such a fundamental challenge to an institution that it creates a set of problems arising from feelings of being devalued. If those who live and work in institutions largely believe that what happens in them is worthwhile and good, the introduction of an ethical audit which challenges these assumptions may well be seen as an insult to their integrity. Responses could range from extensive efforts to justify existing practices to a more fundamental impact on the entire ethos of care. Perhaps this may serve to indicate the value of self-audit, in much the same way as we are beginning to recognise the importance of self-regulation.

Thus, whether practice in institutions is 'good' or 'bad', an ethical audit can have unexpected effects which can arise because of the nature of the institution and the nature of care. This is not to say that these effects will not be felt in other types of organisation with different activities, but it does suggest that digging up the values of an institution is something that must be done carefully. Exactly how carefully, and what form this care should take, is something that needs to be worked out as this approach to audit is developed further.

In debates about business ethics, some strategies and models have been outlined. Wilson (1993), for example, has developed a model of ethical management which takes the ethical audit as a starting point. The results are translated into organisational mission statements and charters and codes. This process is not simply about carrying out an ethical opinion poll and then going with the majority view, but needs to be based on coherent and credible general moral principles. Wilson also points out that without an action plan, such audit and mission statement writing initiatives are likely to be ineffective in changing anything in an organisation. Part of an action plan might involve the creation of an ethics committee, which would monitor activity, oversee debates and the development of codes of practice, carry out ethics training, and provide a forum for support, advice and debate. Wilson argued that the training and education element of the action plan is particularly important if debate is to be informed and the organisation is to develop awareness of ethical issues.

## PERSONAL/PROFESSIONAL

Discussions about practice, and how it can be evaluated, often include two basic premises. First, the way in which practice is evaluated should be mainly about outcomes. In other words, while the processes involved in practice are of interest, the primary focus is on the impact or effect it has: this, by and large, is usually on others apart from the practitioner – it is on clients, colleagues or the wider organisation. Second, discussions of evaluation often assume that the evaluation is carried out by someone other than the practitioner – a colleague, client or manager. This may be on the grounds of 'objectivity', in that ideas about people evaluating their own practice carry a suspicion that they might just see and report what they want to see.

Aside from these externally derived and outcomes-based models, there are some ideas about self-evaluation which include processes that can be gathered together from the literature on practice, particularly in practitioner education. Perhaps the most widely known set of ideas are those which come under the heading 'reflective practice'. The prime exponent of this concept is Schon (1983, 1987) who provided a description of how professionals reflect on the problems that they face in their practice, and argued that this was through a process of utilising theories gained from experience, rather than the simple adherence to abstract rules or theories. Notions of reflective practice, however, focus on problem-solving where the problems are technical: how to do or achieve something. Thus, while reflective practice may be internal, it is still largely outcomes-driven and not about the ethical basis of practice processes.

Nonetheless, ideas about the way in which practitioners reflect are useful, in that they distinguish between abstract formulations of how care should happen, the official version, and experientially based theories built up over time by individual practitioners. Transferring this observation to the use and development of ethical principles in practice, a parallel process could be expected. In other words, while there might be a range of public ethics, mission statements and the like, which stipulate rules of conduct, practitioners may draw on a range of informally acquired ethics derived from experience. These experiential ethics may well have more resonance with practitioners than the rules of the institution and, as we discussed in Chapter 7, there is a view that this is the right way for things to be – that personal morality is more genuine and valid than institutional codes.

The problem with personal, individual ethics, however, is that we cannot compare them with institutional ethics, or at least we have not had a history of doing so. That is partly what the ethical audit does, but it relies on the assumption that eliciting people's ethical positions is a relatively unproblematic process. If experiential knowledge, however, is as difficult to elicit as many have argued, then experiential ethics are likely to be even more problematic. As values become tacit, whereby people cannot say what their principles are, or how they arrived at them, then reflecting on them becomes more difficult.

Following this line of argument directs us to the idea that for there to be some sort of ethical reflection, there needs to be some direction given to practitioners, in training, education or practice. Steadman *et al.* (1994), in a study about how to incorporate ethics into occupational standards, identified a set of skills that practitioners need to have. They also identified four sets of values which impact on practice ethics: legal values, professional values, individual values and the values of the employer. Professionals, they argue, need to be able to evaluate and judge the type of ethical question they are dealing with, and how it is viewed from each of these value positions. Sets of values may conflict where, for example, a professional set of ethics conflicts with those of an individual practitioner, and practitioners need to develop skills to resolve these differences. Steadman *et al.* also argued that some sets of values are so embedded in practice that it is difficult for practitioners to identify them clearly.

There are a number of professional ethics texts that explore these dilemmas in great depth, and some of them include a discussion on frameworks for reflecting on ethical questions (for an overview see Seedhouse, 1988). These are often, however, questions of the 'dramatic ethics' type – around acute dilemmas in care, or specific incidents. While these texts are useful in highlighting and exemplifying some practice dilemmas, there are also questions to be asked about everyday practice. Questions could be asked, for example, about practices such as buying clothes for residents without them being involved. This does not seem quite such a crucial issue as questions about euthanasia or informed consent, but in many ways mundane questions are more important simply because of their undramatic nature – they are about issues that everyone takes for granted.

Seedhouse provides an example of a way of reflecting on ethical aspects of practice in his 'ethical grid'. In this grid, he identifies a range of different aspects which must be taken into account in making an ethical decision, for example professional goals and client preferences, along with considerations of long- and short-term implications of the decision. While Seedhouse's grid is certainly inclusive, as it incorporates a wide range of issues, it is presented as an aid to decision-making and this is portrayed as a discrete episode. As with many frameworks for professional ethics, the discussions that surround them or the way that they are illustrated seem to centre on clearly defined problems or dilemmas. Typically, the readers are presented with a vignette, where there is a dilemma or issue clearly defined, then they are asked to apply the framework and see where it takes them. Applying such frameworks outside the confines of a decision-making episode, and using them to develop firm principles as a basis for ongoing care is not impossible, but it is not always demonstrated clearly in these texts. If we think of ethical reflection in practice as being not just about one-off decisions but about developing consistent principled approaches to care, then the usefulness of these frameworks becomes limited without further development. Ethical frameworks need to look more explicitly at enduring values, at how they shape care, and how they can be examined and debated.

Henry (1995) outlines an exercise for prioritising values, which goes some way towards such an examination. The exercise also has potential for looking at the range of priorities that different people have and the differences that there might be between organisationally espoused values and the values of individuals within it. Henry gives two lists: the first is a list of policies and procedures, such as equal opportunities policy or organisational targets, and the second is a list of values, for example loyalty and beneficence. These lists represent what Henry describes as issues and values frequently identified as important to organisational culture. The exercise consists of taking different perspectives within the organisation, say as manager or care assistant, and arranging the items on the two lists according to the priority that you think that that person would give to them. Henry also suggests that this might be useful to do as a group exercise, to explore differences in work teams.

What this exercise does is highlight possible differences in values across people in organisations. For example, it may be that the values of loyalty are prioritised by managers but not by others, who may give higher priority to the values of fairness and justice. This difference clearly points to something beyond individual personal values, something about the organisation and how it operates. While this is not necessarily a huge problem if the values of people in different roles are different, the potential is there for a number of problems to occur when values are brought into conflict. If, for example, in the interests of fairness, care workers behave in ways which are seen to be disloyal, say, for example by admitting to a client that their service was at fault (and thus opening the way for a claim for compensation against the organisation), there is scope for huge conflicts.

One obvious area in which there can be conflicts of values is between those who work in institutions – the staff, and those who live there – the service-users. Carrying out an exercise like that proposed by Henry may well be extended to the clients of the organisation, and arguably should be in the interests of comprehensive evaluation. Indeed, not to include service-users seems to confound the entire purpose of an ethical audit. Looking to see how service-users prioritise values, say, for example honesty, and how staff do so would be an instructive exercise that could form the basis of organisational change.

## CHALLENGES OF AN ETHICS-BASED APPROACH

We have focused on notions of ethical audit at both an organisational and an individual level. Whereas most evaluations of practice and provision focus on observable outcomes, ethical evaluations need to centre on processes, and need to take pains to elicit non-observable aspects of provision: not just what people do, but why they do it. Separating out the organisational and the individual, however, is a difficult task, as the two are closely linked. Individuals may adhere to a set of values which originate from institutional policies rather than from their own personal reflection, and institutional values may be shaped by the values of those that live and work there.

Nevertheless, making this distinction is a useful exercise in the way that it can identify challenges to an assumed consensus. Where there are differences in values within and between groups, however, it may not be enough to sit back and remark on how interesting this difference is. The purpose of the evaluation should be to move things on and not simply observe. In this sense, an ethical evaluation is only an initial step in practice development, and not an end in itself. Identifying values and principles of care, and the extent to which they are shared, forms a basis for debates on how these values can be operationalised and how differences can be resolved, but in itself it does not resolve these questions. From this point, therefore, it becomes necessary to construct a framework for developing an approach to the ethical audit. To have utility, such an approach requires both structure and flexibility: structure to enable implementation, and flexibility to ensure that local needs and conditions can be met. In the concluding section of this chapter we endeavour to integrate key themes and processes with a view to promoting just such an approach.

## Summary

Our purpose in writing has been first to draw attention to the huge range of literature, together with the many and varied experiences of care that it reflects, which exist concerning institutional care. Our purpose has also been to apply the lessons of that literature to our concept of 'opening up' institutions to a values-based and practice-driven scrutiny which has a very explicit agenda for change. We have demonstrated that none of us is able to claim that institutional life has not been, is not, or will not be, part of our personal experience. We have articulated our firm belief as to the vital utility of institutional care and its continuing, merited, place in the inventory of available facilities. We have also explored a great number of different perspectives and it is not our intention in this final chapter to attempt to summarise them all. To do so would merely serve to beg the question as to why it was necessary to present the detail in the first instance. Our response to such a question would be that we see the detail in the material as central to gaining an understanding into this world with which we are all so centrally concerned. It is an understanding which is grounded in the everyday activities of institutional life, but which locates those activities within a conceptualising framework. It is also an understanding which clearly locates the responsibilities for what transpires within those settings firmly with all concerned with them. To paraphrase Donabedian's observation, which we cited earlier (in Phaneuf, 1976), if the roles of those who work within the residential social and health care settings are to be seen as substantive activities located within a mature professional context, then self-regulation of activity is an imperative. We would add that we believe that the case for the inclusion of a user-perspective imperative is incontrovertible.

Thus, our final task is to tease out the key themes to present as a basis for developing a process of ethical audit. Some of the regulatory models which we have examined have been generalised, or have been developed to serve externalised purposes, whatever their rationale or justification might be. Yet others have been founded in complex and detailed technical protocols, often derived from clinical practice. When we examined audit methodology we discovered a similar variety. We have no wish to replicate such approaches as a model for ourselves and we acknowledge that any setting would require a variety of instruments to serve a variety of purposes. However, what we wish to do, recognising that each care environment is unique in some respects whilst sharing common practices and understandings with others, is to present a synopsis of the themes which emerged during our exploration of audit methodology, with a view to encouraging practitioners, service-users, researchers and students to examine their own position in relation to their own experiences. We hope that the progress we have made in synthesising this material might serve as a basis for further practice development. Therefore, we propose the following inventories, not as recommendations to be routinely followed, but as accessible ideas which have all been explored within the previous chapters and which might be used as a basis for initiating an ethically-oriented review of practice within any institutional setting.

## AN AUDIT SHOULD:

- be cyclical, including an action stage and loop-back process;
- be rigorous and exhaustive;
- be inclusive of all stakeholders;
- be both inward and outward looking, i.e. connect with wider societal perspectives;
- be self-regulatory;
- embrace the notion of self-audit;
- be conscious of the impact of the processes of opening-up care at both institutional/organisational levels and practice/individual levels;
- consider its extent;
- be flexible.

## TO BE ETHICAL AN AUDIT SHOULD:

- not be imposed, but be a consensual process;
- prioritise the issues and values-base of the resident as service-user;
- be clear that its primary purpose is to contribute to good practice;
- develop proposals for making and implementing improvement;
- be primarily concerned with the context of good practice;
- embrace stakeholder participation in development and implementation;
- be open and explicit;
- ensure that its style is not antithetical to the development and maintenance of good practice;
- avoid reification of the 'institution';
- acknowledge that behaviour and values are owned personally as well as collectively;
- be actively associated with other forms of documentation, e.g. mission statements;
- identify, and be based in coherent, credible general moral principles;
- acknowledge the contribution of moral philosophy in thinking about values;
- investigate the operation of values within the institution and how they are manifested in practice;
- consider how difficult ethical practice issues can be raised anonymously;
- be conscious of sensitivities;
- avoid being coercive or punitive;
- provide scope for personal and collective reflexivity;
- address the issue of personal morality versus institutionalised codes;
- address the possibility of the 'corruption' of care through an application of Wardhaugh and Wilding's eight propositions (Allott and Robb, 1998) (see Chapter 3).

## CONCLUSIONS

It is axiomatic that no ethical audit can be initiated until a consensus to do so exists and mechanisms are identified for so doing. There are, therefore, prerequisites for progress which cannot, in the light of our trawl of the literature, be taken for granted. We cannot prescribe in this respect, but we emphasise our earlier comment that we all must bear some responsibility for bringing about conditions which will enable progress to be made. That is not to ignore naïvely the fact that different players will have different levels of power and influence, or that some settings will offer an open door whilst others may be well and firmly bolted. However, not to raise the possibility of progress abdicates all responsibility to the grim spectres which we have identified only too clearly and must avoid. There are also other macro issues, such as the question of how to incorporate ethics more effectively into occupational standards, or how to identify relevant skills which practitioners need and incorporate them into professional training, learning and education programmes. That responsibility lies firmly with those of us who are involved in these areas. We do not underestimate the levels of change which might be required, or the difficulty of the proposed task. Nevertheless, in the quest to achieve principled practice, we have both a moral duty and a professional obligation to take this process forward.

# Bibliography

Adams R, Dominelli L and Payne M (eds) (1998) *Social Work: Themes, Issues and Critical Debates*. London, Macmillan

Aichorn A (1951) *Wayward Youth*. New York, Imago

Ainsworth F and Fulcher L (1981) *Group Care for Children*. London, Tavistock

Allen J (1995) *Surviving the Registration and Inspection Process: A Guide for Care Home Owners and Managers*. London, Pitman Publishing

Allott M and Robb M (eds) (1998) *Understanding Health and Social Care: An Introductory Reader*. London, Sage/Open University, pp. 212–29

Audit Commission (1985) *Capital Expenditure Controls in Local Government in England*. London, HMSO

Audit Commission (1986) *Making a Reality of Community Care*. London, HMSO

Aymer C (1992) *Women in Residential Work: Dilemmas and Ambiguities*. London, Routledge

Baglee C (1971) *The Holy Jesus Hospital*. Newcastle, F. Graham

Baker D (1978) Attitudes of Nurses to the Care of the Elderly. Unpublished PhD thesis, Manchester University

Balbernie R (1966) *Residential Work With Children*. London, Pergamon

Baldwin N, Harris J and Kelly D. Institutionalisation: why blame the institution? *Ageing and Society* 1993, 13(1), 69–81

Bennett M, Smith E and Millard P (1995) The Right Person? The Right Place? The Right Time? Unpublished research report. London, SELHCA

Berridge D (1985) *Children's Homes*. Oxford, Blackwell

Biggs S, Phillipson C and Kingston P (1995) *Elder Abuse in Perspective*. Buckingham, Open University Press

Bion W (1961) *Experiences in Groups*. London, Tavistock Publications

Bowlby J (1953) *Child Care and the Growth of Love*. London, Penguin

Bridgeland M (1971) *Pioneer Work With Maladjusted Children*. London, Staples

Burgner T (1996) *The Regulation and Inspection of Social Services*. London, Department of Health

Burlingham D and Freud A (1944) *Infants Without Families*. London, Allen and Unwin

Burns T and Stalker GM (1961) *The Management of Innovation*. London, Tavistock

Burton J (1993) *The Handbook of Residential Care*. London, Routledge

Cadbury G (1938) *Young Offenders Yesterday and Today*. London, Allen and Unwin

Campbell G (1995) Language and ethics. In Henry C (ed.) *Professional Ethics and Organisational Change*. London, Arnold, pp. 31–44

Care Centre for Policy on Ageing (1984) *Home Life. A Code of Practice for Residential Care: The Avebury Report*. London, CCPA

Care Centre for Policy on Ageing (1996) *A Better Home Life. A Code of Practice for Residential and Nursing Homes*. London, CCPA

Carlebach J (1970) *Caring for Troubled Children*. London, Routledge and Kegan Paul

Chartered Institute of Public Finance and Accountancy (1975) *1975–76 Estimates*. London, Personal Social Services Statistics CIPFA

Clarke M (1978) Getting through the work. In Dingwall R and Macintosh J (eds) *Readings in the Sociology of Nursing*. Edinburgh, Churchill Livingstone

Clough R (1981) *Old Age Homes*. London, Allen and Unwin

Clough R (1988) *Living Away From Home.* Bristol Papers in Applied Social Studies no. 4, University of Bristol

Cohen AP (1989) *The Symbolic Construction of Community.* London, Routledge

*Collins English Dictionary* (3rd edn) (1991) Glasgow, Harper Collins

Collopy BJ. Autonomy in long term care: some crucial distinctions. *Gerontologist*, 1988, 28(suppl.), 10–17

Coulshed V (1990) *Management in Social Work.* Basingstoke, Macmillan Education

Courtioux M, Davies Jones H, Kalcher J, Steinhauser W, Tuggenher H and Waaldijk K (1981) *The Social Pedagogue in Europe: Living with Others as a Profession.* Zurich, Federation Internationale des Communautes Educatives

Cowie LW (1973) *A Dictionary of British Social History.* London, Bell

Crosby P (1979) *Quality Is Free: The Art of Making Quality Certain.* London, McGraw-Hill

Davies M (ed.) (1997) *The Blackwell Companion to Social Work.* Oxford, Blackwell Publishers

Day P, Klein R and Redmayne S (1996) *Why Regulate: Regulating Residential Care for Elderly People.* Bristol, The Policy Press

De Board R 1990 *The Psycho Analysis of Organisations: A Psychoanalytic Approach to Behaviour in Groups and Organisations.* London, Routledge

Department of Health (1989) *Working for Patients.* Medical audit: NHS review working paper no. 6. London, HMSO

Department of Health White Paper (1989) *Caring for People.* London, Department of Health

Department of Health (1991) *Inspecting for Quality: Guidance on Practice for Inspection Units in Social Services Departments and Other Agencies.* London, HMSO

Department of Health (1993) *The Inspection of the Complaints Procedures in Local Authority Social Services Departments.* London, HMSO

Department of Health (1998) *Modernising Social Services.* London, The Stationery Office, Cmnd 4169

Donabedian A (1980) *Exploration in Quality Assessment and Monitoring.* Volume 1: *Definition of Quality and Approaches to it.* University of Michigan, Health Administration Press

Doyal L. Women, health and the sexual division of labour: a case study of the women's health movement in Britain. *Critical Social Policy*, 1983, 7, 21–33

Duncan P. Ethical audit: should it concern health promoters? *Journal of The Institute of Health Education*, 1995, 33(3). (Abstract can be found on the Internet at www.salford.ac.uk/healthSci/jihe33_3.htm)

Dworkin R (1978) *Taking Rights Seriously.* London, Duckworth

Ellis R (ed.) (1988) *Competence and Quality Assurance in the Caring Professions.* Beckenham, Croom Helm

Erikson E (1959) *Identity and the Life Cycle.* New York, International Universities Press

Evers HK. The creation of patients' careers in geriatric wards: aspects of policy and practice. *Social Science and Medicine*, 1981, 15(A), 581–8

Fayol H (1841–1925) (1988) *General Industrial Management.* London, Pitman

Forrest R. The meaning of home ownership. *Society and Space*, 1983, 1, 205–16

Foucault M (1965) *Madness and Civilisation* (translated by R Howard). New York, Pantheon

Fox NJ (1993) *Postmodernism, Sociology and Health.* Buckingham, Open University Press

Frazer E, Hornsby J and Lovibond S (1992) *Ethics: A Feminist Reader.* Oxford, Blackwell

Freidson E (1994) *Professionalism Reborn: Theory, Prophecy and Policy.* Cambridge, Polity Press

Fulcher L and Ainsworth F (1985) *Group Care Practice With Children.* London, Tavistock

Gillon R (1986) *Philosophical Medical Ethics*. Chichester, Wiley

Glouberman S (1990) *Keepers: Inside Stories from Total Institutions*. London, Kings Fund Publishing Office

Goffman E (1961) *Asylums: Essays on the Social Situation of Mental Patients and Other Inmates*. London, Pelican

Griffiths Report (1988) *Community Care, Agenda for Action*. London, HMSO

Gubrium JF (1975) *Living and Dying at Murray Manor*. New York, St Martin's Press

Gubrium JF (1993) *Speaking of Life: Horizons of Meaning for Nursing Home Residents*. New York, Aldine

Gutheil IA. Intimacy in nursing home friendships. *Journal of Gerontological Social Work*, 1991, 17(1/2), 59–73

Hall P (1st edn 1952; 8th edn 1971; 10th edn 1983) *Social Services of England and Wales*. London, Routledge and Kegan Paul

Handy C (1989) *The Age of Unreason*. London, Hutchinson

Handy C (1994) *The Empty Raincoat: Making Sense of the Future*. London, Hutchinson

Henry C (ed.) (1995) *Professional Ethics and Organisational Change in Education and Health*. London, Arnold

Heyman R (ed.) (1998) *Risk, Health and Healthcare: A Qualitative Approach*. London, Arnold

Heywood J (1965) *Children in Care*. London, Routledge and Kegan Paul

Higginson I (1992) *Quality, Standards, Organisational and Clinical Audit for Hospice and Palliative Care Services*. Occasional Paper 2. London, National Council for Hospice and Specialist Palliative Care Services

Hochschild A (1983) *The Managed Heart: Commercialisation of Human Feeling*. Berkeley, University of California Press

Hoghughi M (1978) *Troubled and Troublesome*. London, Burnett

Howard J (1777; 1929 reprint) *The State of the Prisons in England and Wales*. London, Dent

Hugman R (1991) *Power in Caring Professions*. Basingstoke, Macmillan

Illich I (1971) *Celebration of Awareness*. New York, Calder and Boyers

Irvine J and Gertig P. Brave new world: social workers' perceptions of care management. *Practice*, 1998, 10(2), 5–14

Jack R (1998) *Residential Versus Community Care: The Role of Institutions in Welfare Provision*. Basingstoke, Macmillan Press

Jones H (1979) *The Residential Community*. London, Routledge and Kegan Paul

Jones K and Fowles AJ (1984) *Ideas on Institutions: Analysing the Literature on Long-Term Care and Custody*. London, Routledge and Kegan Paul

Jones M (1973) *Beyond the Therapeutic Community*. Yale, University of Yale Press

Kahan B (1994) *Growing Up in Groups*. London, HMSO/National Institute for Social Work

Kellaher L (1992) *Inside Quality Assurance Action Pack*. University of North London, Centre for Environmental Social Studies in Ageing

Kelly MP and May D. Good and bad patients: a review of the literature and a theoretical critique. *Journal of Advanced Nursing*, 1982, 7(2), 147–57

Kerruish A and Smith H (1993) *Developing Quality Residential Care: A User Led Approach*. Harlow, Longman

Lasson I (1981) *Where's My Mum?* London, Pepar

Lawton A and Rose A (1994) *Organisation and Management in the Public Sector*. London, Pitman

Le Grand J (1990) *Quasi-Markets and Social Policy*. University of Bristol, School for Advanced Urban Studies

Likert R (1987) *New Patterns of Management*. London, Garland

Lock D (1990) *Handbook of Quality Management*. London, Gower

Mallinson I (1995) *Keyworking in Social Care: A Structured Approach to Provision*. London, Whiting & Birch/SCA (Education)

Malthus TR (1766–1834) (1966) *An Essay on the Principle of Population*. London, Routledge

Mann T (1996) *Clinical Audit in the NHS: Using Clinical Audit in the NHS, a Position Statement*. Leeds, NHS Executive

Manton J (1976) *Mary Carpenter and the Children of the Streets*. London, Heineman Educational Books

Maslow AH (1970) *Motivation and Personality*, 2nd edn. London, Harper Row

Mayhew H (1967) *London Labour and the London Poor*. London, Frank Cass

McCord N (1979) *North East England, The Region's Development 1760–1960*. London, Batsford Academic

McGregor D (1985) *The Human Side of Enterprise*, 25th anniversary printing edn. London, McGraw-Hill

McNay M (1992) In Langan M and Day L (eds) *Women, Oppression and Social Work*. London, Routledge

Menzies I (1960) *The Functioning of Social Systems as a Defence Against Anxiety*. London, Tavistock

Midgley M (1981) *Heart and Mind: The Varieties of Moral Experience*. London, Methuen

Miller EJ and Gwynne GV (1972) *A Life Apart*. London, Tavistock

Millham S, Bullock R and Cherrett P (1975) *After Grace – Teeth*. London, Human Context Books

Moos RH (1974) *Evaluating Treatment Environments: A Social Ecological Approach*. New York, Wiley

Moos RH (1987) *The Social Climate Scales: A User's Guide*. California, Consulting Psychologists Press

Moos RH and Lemke S (1994) *Group Residences for Older Adults: Physical Features, Policies, and Social Climate*. New York, Oxford University Press

Neill AS (1970) *Summerhill*. London, Penguin

Nocon A and Qureshi H (1996) *Outcomes of Community Care for Users and Carers*. Buckingham, Open University Press

O'Kell S (1995) *Care Standards in the Residential Care Sector: Quality and Qualifications*. York, Joseph Rowntree Foundation

Olafson FA (1973) *Ethics and Twentieth Century Thought*. Hemel Hempstead, Prentice-Hall

Øvretveit H, Matthias P and Thompson T (1997) *Interprofessional Working for Health and Social Care*. London, Macmillan

Oxley GW (1974) *Poor Relief in England and Wales 1601–1834*. Newton Abbot, David and Charles

Parker I, Georgaca E, Harper D, McLaughlin T and Stowell-Smith M (1995) *Deconstructing Psychopathology*. London, Sage

Paton HR (1948) *Groundwork of the Metaphysics of Morals*. London, Hutchinson

Peace S, Kellaher L and Willcocks D (1997) *Re-Evaluating Residential Care*. Buckingham, Open University Press

Peters T (1987) *Thriving on Chaos*. New York, Harper and Row

Peters TJ and Waterman RH Jr (1982) *In Search of Excellence. Lessons from America's Best-Run Companies*. New York, Harper and Row

Phaneuf MC (1976) . *The Nursing Audit: Self-Regulation in Nursing Practice*. New York, Appleton-Century-Crofts

Pinchbeck I and Hewitt M (1973) *Children in English Society*, vols 1 and 2. London, Routledge and Kegan Paul

Polsky HW (1962) *Cottage Six*. New York, Russell Sage

Porter S. Real bodies, real needs: a critique of the application of Foucault's philosophy to nursing. *Social Sciences in Health*, 1996, 2(4), 218–27

Raynes NV, Wright K, Shiell A and Pettipher C (1994) *The Cost and Quality of Community Residential Care*. London, David Fulton Publishers

Reed J and Ground I (1997) *Philosophy for Nursing*. London, Arnold

Reed J and Payton V (1996) *Working to Create Continuity: Older People Managing the Move to the Care Home Setting*. University of Newcastle upon Tyne, Centre for Health Services Research, Report no. 76

Rose M (1990) *Healing Hurt Minds: the Peper Harow Experience*. London, Tavistock

Rose M (1997) *Transforming Hate to Love*. London, Routledge

Rousseau JJ (1968) *Social Contract*. Harmondsworth, Penguin

Royal Society (1992) *Risk: Analysis, Perception and Management: Report of a Royal Society Study Group*. London, The Royal Society

Sabine G (1973) *A History of Political Theory*, 4th edn (revised by Thorson TL). London, Harrap

Schon D (1983) *The Reflective Practitioner: How Professionals Think in Action*. New York, Basic Books

Schon D (1987) *Educating the Reflective Practitioner: Towards a New Design for Teaching and Learning in the Professions*. San Francisco, Jossey-Bass

Scull AT (1979) *Museums of Madness*. London, Penguin

Scull AT (1981) *Madhouses, Mad Doctors, and Madmen*. London, Athlone

Seedhouse D (1988) *Ethics: The Heart of Health Care*. Chichester, John Wiley

Shotter J (1993) *Cultural Politics of Everyday Life*. Buckingham, Open University Press

Sixsmith J. The meaning of home: an exploratory study of environmental experience. *Journal of Environmental Psychology*, 1986, 6, 281–98

Smith P (1992) *The Emotional Labour of Nursing*. London, Macmillan

Staffordshire County Council (1991) *The Pindown Experience and the Protection of Children: The Report of the Staffordshire Child Care Inquiry 1990*. Staffordshire, Staffordshire County Council

Stanley D (1978) Residential Child Care: A Rationale for Practice. Unpublished BPhil dissertation, University of Newcastle upon Tyne

Stanley D (1989) The Anatomy of Group Care. Unpublished PhD thesis, University of Newcastle upon Tyne

Steadman S, Eraut M, Cole G and Marquand L (1994) *Ethics in Occupational Standards*. Sheffield, Sheffield Employment Department, Methods Strategy Unit

Stewart G and Tutt N (1987) *Children in Custody*. London, Avebury (Gower)

Szasz TS (1961) *The Myth of Mental Illness: Foundations of a Theory of Personal Conduct*. New York, Dell

Tester S (1996) *Community Care for Older People: A Comparative Perspective*. London, Macmillan

Tizard J, Sinclair I and Clarke RVG (eds) (1975) *Varieties of Residential Experience*. London, Routledge

Tomlinson D and Carrier J (eds) (1996) *Asylum in the Community*. London, Routledge

Townsend P (1962) *The Last Refuge: A Survey of Residential Institutions and Homes for the Aged in England and Wales*. London, Routledge and Kegan Paul

Utting W (1991) *Children in the Public Care*. London, HMSO

Wagner Report (1988) Part 1. *Residential Care: A Positive Choice*. London, HMSO

Wagner Report (1988) Part 2. *Residential Care: The Research Reviewed*. London, HMSO

Walton R and Elliott D (1980) *Residential Care, A Reader in Current Theory and Practice.* Oxford, Pergamon

Warnock M (ed.) (1962) *Utilitarianism.* London, Fontana

Weber M (1864–1920) (1985) The *Protestant Ethic and the Spirit of Capitalism* (translated by Talcott Parsons). London, Unwin

Wilkins D and Hughes B. Residential care of elderly people: the consumers' view. *Ageing and Society,* 1987, 7, 175–201

Williams Report (1967) *Caring for People, Staff in Residential Homes.* London, Allen and Unwin

Wills D (1971) *Spare the Child.* London, Penguin

Wilmot S (1997) *The Ethics of Community* Care. London, Cassell

Wilson A. Translating corporate values into business behaviour. *Business Ethics: A European Review,* 1993, 2(2), 103–5

Wilson J (1997) *Integrated Care Management: The Path to Success?* Oxford, Butterworth Heinemann

Wittgenstein L (1958) *Philosophical Investigations,* 2nd edn. (translated by Anscombe GEM). Oxford, Blackwell

Witz A (1992) *Patriarchy and Professions.* London, Routledge

Wolins M (ed.) (1974) *Successful Group Care.* Chicago, Aldine

Wolins M and Wozner Y (1982) *Revitalizing Residential Settings.* San Francisco, Jossey-Bass

Youll PJ and McCourt-Perring C (1993) *Raising Voices: Ensuring Quality in Residential Care.* London, HMSO

# Index